THE OFFICIAL PATIENT'S SOURCEBOOK on

MERKEL CELL CARCINOMA

JAMES N. PARKER, M.D.
AND PHILIP M. PARKER, PH.D., EDITORS

ICON Health Publications
ICON Group International, Inc.
4370 La Jolla Village Drive, 4th Floor
San Diego, CA 92122 USA

Copyright ©2002 by ICON Group International, Inc.

Copyright ©2002 by ICON Group International, Inc. All rights reserved. This book is protected by copyright. No part of it may be reproduced, stored in a retrieval system, or transmitted in any form or by any means, electronic, mechanical, photocopying, recording or otherwise, without written permission from the publisher.

Printed in the United States of America.

Last digit indicates print number: 10 9 8 7 6 4 5 3 2 1

Publisher, Health Care: Tiffany LaRochelle
Editor(s): James Parker, M.D., Philip Parker, Ph.D.

Publisher's note: The ideas, procedures, and suggestions contained in this book are not intended as a substitute for consultation with your physician. All matters regarding your health require medical supervision. As new medical or scientific information becomes available from academic and clinical research, recommended treatments and drug therapies may undergo changes. The authors, editors, and publisher have attempted to make the information in this book up to date and accurate in accord with accepted standards at the time of publication. The authors, editors, and publisher are not responsible for errors or omissions or for consequences from application of the book, and make no warranty, expressed or implied, in regard to the contents of this book. Any practice described in this book should be applied by the reader in accordance with professional standards of care used in regard to the unique circumstances that may apply in each situation, in close consultation with a qualified physician. The reader is advised to always check product information (package inserts) for changes and new information regarding dose and contraindications before taking any drug or pharmacological product. Caution is especially urged when using new or infrequently ordered drugs, herbal remedies, vitamins and supplements, alternative therapies, complementary therapies and medicines, and integrative medical treatments.

Cataloging-in-Publication Data

Parker, James N., 1961-
Parker, Philip M., 1960-

The Official Patient's Sourcebook on Merkel Cell Carcinoma: A Revised and Updated Directory for the Internet Age/James N. Parker and Philip M. Parker, editors
    p.   cm.
Includes bibliographical references, glossary and index.
ISBN: 0-597-83478-4
1. Merkel Cell Carcinoma-Popular works.   I. Title.

Disclaimer

This publication is not intended to be used for the diagnosis or treatment of a health problem or as a substitute for consultation with licensed medical professionals. It is sold with the understanding that the publisher, editors, and authors are not engaging in the rendering of medical, psychological, financial, legal, or other professional services.

References to any entity, product, service, or source of information that may be contained in this publication should not be considered an endorsement, either direct or implied, by the publisher, editors or authors. ICON Group International, Inc., the editors, or the authors are not responsible for the content of any Web pages nor publications referenced in this publication.

Copyright Notice

If a physician wishes to copy limited passages from this sourcebook for patient use, this right is automatically granted without written permission from ICON Group International, Inc. (ICON Group). However, all of ICON Group publications are copyrighted. With exception to the above, copying our publications in whole or in part, for whatever reason, is a violation of copyright laws and can lead to penalties and fines. Should you want to copy tables, graphs or other materials, please contact us to request permission (e-mail: iconedit@san.rr.com). ICON Group often grants permission for very limited reproduction of our publications for internal use, press releases, and academic research. Such reproduction requires confirmed permission from ICON Group International Inc. **The disclaimer above must accompany all reproductions, in whole or in part, of this sourcebook.**

Dedication

To the healthcare professionals dedicating their time and efforts to the study of merkel cell carcinoma.

Acknowledgements

The collective knowledge generated from academic and applied research summarized in various references has been critical in the creation of this sourcebook which is best viewed as a comprehensive compilation and collection of information prepared by various official agencies which directly or indirectly are dedicated to merkel cell carcinoma. All of the *Official Patient's Sourcebooks* draw from various agencies and institutions associated with the United States Department of Health and Human Services, and in particular, the Office of the Secretary of Health and Human Services (OS), the Administration for Children and Families (ACF), the Administration on Aging (AOA), the Agency for Healthcare Research and Quality (AHRQ), the Agency for Toxic Substances and Disease Registry (ATSDR), the Centers for Disease Control and Prevention (CDC), the Food and Drug Administration (FDA), the Healthcare Financing Administration (HCFA), the Health Resources and Services Administration (HRSA), the Indian Health Service (IHS), the institutions of the National Institutes of Health (NIH), the Program Support Center (PSC), and the Substance Abuse and Mental Health Services Administration (SAMHSA). In addition to these sources, information gathered from the National Library of Medicine, the United States Patent Office, the European Union, and their related organizations has been invaluable in the creation of this sourcebook. Some of the work represented was financially supported by the Research and Development Committee at INSEAD. This support is gratefully acknowledged. Finally, special thanks are owed to Tiffany LaRochelle for her excellent editorial support.

About the Editors

James N. Parker, M.D.

Dr. James N. Parker received his Bachelor of Science degree in Psychobiology from the University of California, Riverside and his M.D. from the University of California, San Diego. In addition to authoring numerous research publications, he has lectured at various academic institutions. Dr. Parker is the medical editor for the *Official Patient's Sourcebook* series published by ICON Health Publications.

Philip M. Parker, Ph.D.

Philip M. Parker is the Eli Lilly Chair Professor of Innovation, Business and Society at INSEAD (Fontainebleau, France and Singapore). Dr. Parker has also been Professor at the University of California, San Diego and has taught courses at Harvard University, the Hong Kong University of Science and Technology, the Massachusetts Institute of Technology, Stanford University, and UCLA. Dr. Parker is the associate editor for the *Official Patient's Sourcebook* series published by ICON Health Publications.

About ICON Health Publications

In addition to merkel cell carcinoma, *Official Patient's Sourcebooks* are available for he following related topics:

- The Official Patient's Sourcebook on Melanoma
- The Official Patient's Sourcebook on Skin Cancer

To discover more about ICON Health Publications, simply check with your preferred online booksellers, including Barnes & Noble.com and Amazon.com which currently carry all of our titles. Or, feel free to contact us directly for bulk purchases or institutional discounts:

> ICON Group International, Inc.
> 4370 La Jolla Village Drive, Fourth Floor
> San Diego, CA 92122 USA
> Fax: 858-546-4341
> Web site: **www.icongrouponline.com/health**

Table of Contents

INTRODUCTION 1
   Overview 1
   Organization 3
   Scope 3
   Moving Forward 4

PART I: THE ESSENTIALS 7

CHAPTER 1. THE ESSENTIALS ON MERKEL CELL CARCINOMA: GUIDELINES 9
   Overview 9
   What Is Merkel Cell Carcinoma? 11
   Stages of Merkel Cell Carcinoma 12
   How Is Merkel Cell Carcinoma Treated? 12
   Treatment by Stage 14
   To Learn More 15
   About PDQ 16
   More Guideline Sources 17
   Vocabulary Builder 20

CHAPTER 2. SEEKING GUIDANCE 23
   Overview 23
   Associations and Merkel Cell Carcinoma 23
   Finding More Associations 28
   Cancer Support Groups 29
   The Cancer Information Service 31
   Finding Cancer Resources in Your Community 34
   Finding Doctors Who Specialize in Cancer Care 38
   Selecting Your Doctor 40
   Working with Your Doctor 41
   Finding a Cancer Treatment Facility 42
   Additional Cancer Support Information 44
   Vocabulary Builder 45

CHAPTER 3. CLINICAL TRIALS AND MERKEL CELL CARCINOMA 47
   Overview 47
   Recent Trials on Merkel Cell Carcinoma 50
   Benefits and Risks 51
   Clinical Trials and Insurance Coverage 54
   Clinical Trials and Medicare Coverage 57
   Increasing the Likelihood of Insurance Coverage for Trials 58
   If Your Insurance Claim Is Denied after the Trial Has Begun 60
   Government Initiatives to Expand Insurance Coverage for Trials 63
   Keeping Current on Clinical Trials 64

General References..65
Vocabulary Builder..66

PART II: ADDITIONAL RESOURCES AND ADVANCED MATERIAL 67

CHAPTER 4. STUDIES ON MERKEL CELL CARCINOMA......................69
Overview..69
Federally Funded Research on Merkel Cell Carcinoma............................69
E-Journals: PubMed Central..71
The National Library of Medicine: PubMed..72
Vocabulary Builder..90

CHAPTER 5. BOOKS ON MERKEL CELL CARCINOMA.......................95
Overview..95
The National Library of Medicine Book Index...95
Chapters on Merkel Cell Carcinoma..96
General Home References..96
Vocabulary Builder..97

CHAPTER 6. PHYSICIAN GUIDELINES AND DATABASES....................99
Overview..99
NIH Guidelines..99
What Is Merkel Cell Carcinoma?..100
Cellular Classification..101
Stage Information...102
Treatment Option Overview...103
NIH Databases..106
Other Commercial Databases...110
The Genome Project and Merkel Cell Carcinoma..................................111
Specialized References..115
Vocabulary Builder..116

PART III. APPENDICES 117

APPENDIX A. RESEARCHING YOUR MEDICATIONS.......................119
Overview..119
Your Medications: The Basics..120
Learning More about Your Medications..122
Commercial Databases...122
Drug Development and Approval..123
Understanding the Approval Process for New Cancer Drugs................125
The Role of the Federal Drug Administration (FDA)............................125
Getting Drugs to Patients Who Need Them..129
Contraindications and Interactions (Hidden Dangers).........................131
A Final Warning..132
General References...133

Vocabulary Builder *133*
APPENDIX B. RESEARCHING ALTERNATIVE MEDICINE 135
Overview *135*
What Is CAM? *136*
What Are the Domains of Alternative Medicine? *137*
Finding CAM References on Merkel Cell Carcinoma *142*
Additional Web Resources *146*
General References *146*
Vocabulary Builder *148*
APPENDIX C. RESEARCHING NUTRITION 149
Overview *149*
Food and Nutrition: General Principles *150*
Finding Studies on Merkel Cell Carcinoma *154*
Federal Resources on Nutrition *157*
Additional Web Resources *158*
Vocabulary Builder *158*
APPENDIX D. FINDING MEDICAL LIBRARIES 161
Overview *161*
Preparation *161*
Finding a Local Medical Library *162*
Medical Libraries Open to the Public *162*
APPENDIX E. YOUR RIGHTS AND INSURANCE 169
Overview *169*
Your Rights as a Patient *169*
Patient Responsibilities *173*
Choosing an Insurance Plan *174*
Medicare and Medicaid *176*
Financial Assistance for Cancer Care *179*
NORD's Medication Assistance Programs *182*
Additional Resources *183*

ONLINE GLOSSARIES 185
Online Dictionary Directories *186*

MERKEL CELL CARCINOMA GLOSSARY 187
General Dictionaries and Glossaries *198*

INDEX 201

INTRODUCTION

Overview

Dr. C. Everett Koop, former U.S. Surgeon General, once said, "The best prescription is knowledge."[1] The Agency for Healthcare Research and Quality (AHRQ) of the National Institutes of Health (NIH) echoes this view and recommends that every patient incorporate education into the treatment process. According to the AHRQ:

> Finding out more about your condition is a good place to start. By contacting groups that support your condition, visiting your local library, and searching on the Internet, you can find good information to help guide your treatment decisions. Some information may be hard to find — especially if you don't know where to look.[2]

As the AHRQ mentions, finding the right information is not an obvious task. Though many physicians and public officials had thought that the emergence of the Internet would do much to assist patients in obtaining reliable information, in March 2001 the National Institutes of Health issued the following warning:

> The number of Web sites offering health-related resources grows every day. Many sites provide valuable information, while others may have information that is unreliable or misleading.[3]

---

[1] Quotation from **http://www.drkoop.com**.
[2] The Agency for Healthcare Research and Quality (AHRQ): **http://www.ahcpr.gov/consumer/diaginfo.htm**.
[3] Adapted from the NIH, National Cancer Institute (NCI): **http://cancertrials.nci.nih.gov/beyond/evaluating.html**.

Since the late 1990s, physicians have seen a general increase in patient Internet usage rates. Patients frequently enter their doctor's offices with printed Web pages of home remedies in the guise of latest medical research. This scenario is so common that doctors often spend more time dispelling misleading information than guiding patients through sound therapies. *The Official Patient's Sourcebook on Merkel Cell Carcinoma* has been created for patients who have decided to make education and research an integral part of the treatment process. The pages that follow will tell you where and how to look for information covering virtually all topics related to merkel cell carcinoma, from the essentials to the most advanced areas of research.

The title of this book includes the word "official." This reflects the fact that the sourcebook draws from public, academic, government, and peer-reviewed research. Selected readings from various agencies are reproduced to give you some of the latest official information available to date on merkel cell carcinoma.

Given patients' increasing sophistication in using the Internet, abundant references to reliable Internet-based resources are provided throughout this sourcebook. Where possible, guidance is provided on how to obtain free-of-charge, primary research results as well as more detailed information via the Internet. E-book and electronic versions of this sourcebook are fully interactive with each of the Internet sites mentioned (clicking on a hyperlink automatically opens your browser to the site indicated). Hard copy users of this sourcebook can type cited Web addresses directly into their browsers to obtain access to the corresponding sites. Since we are working with ICON Health Publications, hard copy *Sourcebooks* are frequently updated and printed on demand to ensure that the information provided is current.

In addition to extensive references accessible via the Internet, every chapter presents a "Vocabulary Builder." Many health guides offer glossaries of technical or uncommon terms in an appendix. In editing this sourcebook, we have decided to place a smaller glossary within each chapter that covers terms used in that chapter. Given the technical nature of some chapters, you may need to revisit many sections. Building one's vocabulary of medical terms in such a gradual manner has been shown to improve the learning process.

We must emphasize that no sourcebook on merkel cell carcinoma should affirm that a specific diagnostic procedure or treatment discussed in a research study, patent, or doctoral dissertation is "correct" or your best option. This sourcebook is no exception. Each patient is unique. Deciding on appropriate options is always up to the patient in consultation with their physician and healthcare providers.

Organization

This sourcebook is organized into three parts. Part I explores basic techniques to researching merkel cell carcinoma (e.g. finding guidelines on diagnosis, treatments, and prognosis), followed by a number of topics, including information on how to get in touch with organizations, associations, or other patient networks dedicated to merkel cell carcinoma. It also gives you sources of information that can help you find a doctor in your local area specializing in treating merkel cell carcinoma. Collectively, the material presented in Part I is a complete primer on basic research topics for patients with merkel cell carcinoma.

Part II moves on to advanced research dedicated to merkel cell carcinoma. Part II is intended for those willing to invest many hours of hard work and study. It is here that we direct you to the latest scientific and applied research on merkel cell carcinoma. When possible, contact names, links via the Internet, and summaries are provided. It is in Part II where the vocabulary process becomes important as authors publishing advanced research frequently use highly specialized language. In general, every attempt is made to recommend "free-to-use" options.

Part III provides appendices of useful background reading for all patients with merkel cell carcinoma or related disorders. The appendices are dedicated to more pragmatic issues faced by many patients with merkel cell carcinoma. Accessing materials via medical libraries may be the only option for some readers, so a guide is provided for finding local medical libraries which are open to the public. Part III, therefore, focuses on advice that goes beyond the biological and scientific issues facing patients with merkel cell carcinoma.

Scope

While this sourcebook covers merkel cell carcinoma, your doctor, research publications, and specialists may refer to your condition using a variety of terms. Therefore, you should understand that merkel cell carcinoma is often considered a synonym or a condition closely related to the following:

- Merkel Cancer

- Merkel Cell Cancer

For the purposes of this sourcebook, we have attempted to be as inclusive as possible, looking for official information for all of the synonyms relevant to merkel cell carcinoma. You may find it useful to refer to synonyms when accessing databases or interacting with healthcare professionals and medical librarians.

Moving Forward

Since the 1980s, the world has seen a proliferation of healthcare guides covering most illnesses. Some are written by patients or their family members. These generally take a layperson's approach to understanding and coping with an illness or disorder. They can be uplifting, encouraging, and highly supportive. Other guides are authored by physicians or other healthcare providers who have a more clinical outlook. Each of these two styles of guide has its purpose and can be quite useful.

As editors, we have chosen a third route. We have chosen to expose you to as many sources of official and peer-reviewed information as practical, for the purpose of educating you about basic and advanced knowledge as recognized by medical science today. You can think of this sourcebook as your personal Internet age reference librarian.

Why "Internet age"? All too often, patients diagnosed with merkel cell carcinoma will log on to the Internet, type words into a search engine, and receive several Web site listings which are mostly irrelevant or redundant. These patients are left to wonder where the relevant information is, and how to obtain it. Since only the smallest fraction of information dealing with merkel cell carcinoma is even indexed in search engines, a non-systematic approach often leads to frustration and disappointment. With this sourcebook, we hope to direct you to the information you need that you would not likely find using popular Web directories. Beyond Web listings, in many cases we will reproduce brief summaries or abstracts of available reference materials. These abstracts often contain distilled information on topics of discussion.

While we focus on the more scientific aspects of merkel cell carcinoma, there is, of course, the emotional side to consider. Later in the sourcebook, we provide a chapter dedicated to helping you find peer groups and associations that can provide additional support beyond research produced by medical science. We hope that the choices we have made give you the most options available in moving forward. In this way, we wish you the best in your efforts to incorporate this educational approach into your treatment plan.

The Editors

PART I: THE ESSENTIALS

ABOUT PART I

Part I has been edited to give you access to what we feel are "the essentials" on merkel cell carcinoma. The essentials of a disease typically include the definition or description of the disease, a discussion of who it affects, the signs or symptoms associated with the disease, tests or diagnostic procedures that might be specific to the disease, and treatments for the disease. Your doctor or healthcare provider may have already explained the essentials of merkel cell carcinoma to you or even given you a pamphlet or brochure describing merkel cell carcinoma. Now you are searching for more in-depth information. As editors, we have decided, nevertheless, to include a discussion on where to find essential information that can complement what your doctor has already told you. In this section we recommend a process, not a particular Web site or reference book. The process ensures that, as you search the Web, you gain background information in such a way as to maximize your understanding.

CHAPTER 1. THE ESSENTIALS ON MERKEL CELL CARCINOMA: GUIDELINES

Overview

Official agencies, as well as federally funded institutions supported by national grants, frequently publish a variety of guidelines on merkel cell carcinoma. These are typically called "Fact Sheets" or "Guidelines." They can take the form of a brochure, information kit, pamphlet, or flyer. Often they are only a few pages in length. The great advantage of guidelines over other sources is that they are often written with the patient in mind. Since new guidelines on merkel cell carcinoma can appear at any moment and be published by a number of sources, the best approach to finding guidelines is to systematically scan the Internet-based services that post them.

The National Institutes of Health (NIH)[4]

The National Institutes of Health (NIH) is the first place to search for relatively current patient guidelines and fact sheets on merkel cell carcinoma. Originally founded in 1887, the NIH is one of the world's foremost medical research centers and the federal focal point for medical research in the United States. At any given time, the NIH supports some 35,000 research grants at universities, medical schools, and other research and training institutions, both nationally and internationally. The rosters of those who have conducted research or who have received NIH support over the years include the world's most illustrious scientists and physicians. Among them are 97 scientists who have won the Nobel Prize for achievement in medicine.

---

[4] Adapted from the NIH: **http://www.nih.gov/about/NIHoverview.html**.

There is no guarantee that any one Institute will have a guideline on a specific disease, though the National Institutes of Health collectively publish over 600 guidelines for both common and rare diseases. The best way to access NIH guidelines is via the Internet. Although the NIH is organized into many different Institutes and Offices, the following is a list of key Web sites where you are most likely to find NIH clinical guidelines and publications dealing with merkel cell carcinoma and associated conditions:

- Office of the Director (OD); guidelines consolidated across agencies available at **http://www.nih.gov/health/consumer/conkey.htm**

- National Library of Medicine (NLM); extensive encyclopedia (A.D.A.M., Inc.) with guidelines available at **http://www.nlm.nih.gov/medlineplus/healthtopics.html**

- National Cancer Institute (NCI); guidelines available at **http://cancernet.nci.nih.gov/pdq/pdq_treatment.shtml**

Among the above, the National Cancer Institute (NCI) is particularly noteworthy. The NCI coordinates the National Cancer Program, which conducts and supports research, training, health information dissemination, and other programs with respect to the cause, diagnosis, prevention, and treatment of cancer, rehabilitation from cancer, and the continuing care of cancer patients and the families of cancer patients.[5] Specifically, the Institute:

- Supports and coordinates research projects conducted by universities, hospitals, research foundations, and businesses throughout this country and abroad through research grants and cooperative agreements.

- Conducts research in its own laboratories and clinics.

- Supports education and training in fundamental sciences and clinical disciplines for participation in basic and clinical research programs and treatment programs relating to cancer through career awards, training grants, and fellowships.

- Supports research projects in cancer control.

- Supports a national network of cancer centers.

- Collaborates with voluntary organizations and other national and foreign institutions engaged in cancer research and training activities.

- Encourages and coordinates cancer research by industrial concerns where such concerns evidence a particular capability for programmatic research.

- Collects and disseminates information on cancer.

---

[5] This paragraph has been adapted from the NCI: **http://www.nci.nih.gov/**. "Adapted" signifies that a passage has been reproduced exactly or slightly edited for this book.

- Supports construction of laboratories, clinics, and related facilities necessary for cancer research through the award of construction grants.

The NCI, established under the National Cancer Act of 1937, is the Federal Government's principal agency for cancer research and training. The National Cancer Act of 1971 broadened the scope and responsibilities of the NCI and created the National Cancer Program. Over the years, legislative amendments have maintained the NCI authorities and responsibilities and added new information dissemination mandates as well as a requirement to assess the incorporation of state-of-the-art cancer treatments into clinical practice. Information dissemination is made possible through the NCI Online at **www.cancer.gov**. Cancer.gov offers to the public and physicians up-to-date information on the latest cancer research, current and upcoming clinical trials, statistics, research programs, and research funding.

The following patient guideline was recently published by the NCI on merkel cell carcinoma.

What Is Merkel Cell Carcinoma?[6]

Merkel cell carcinoma, also called neuroendocrine cancer of the skin, is a rare type of disease in which malignant (cancer) cells are found on or just beneath the skin and in hair follicles. Merkel cell carcinoma usually appears as firm, painless, shiny lumps of skin. These lumps or tumors can be red, pink, or blue in color and vary in size from less than a quarter of an inch to more than two inches. Merkel cell carcinoma is usually found on the sun-exposed areas of the head, neck, arms, and legs. This type of cancer occurs mostly in whites between 60 and 80 years of age, but it can occur in people of other races and ages as well.

Merkel cell carcinoma grows rapidly and often metastasizes (spreads) to other parts of the body. Even relatively small tumors are capable of metastasizing. When the disease spreads, it tends to spread to the regional (nearby) lymph nodes and may also spread to the liver, bone, lungs, and brain. Lymph nodes are small, bean-shaped structures that are found throughout the body. They produce and store infection-fighting cells.

Treatment of Merkel cell carcinoma depends on the stage of the disease, and the patient's age and overall condition.

---

[6] The following guidelines appeared on the NCI Web site on Aug. 26, 2002. The text was last modified in August 2002. The text has been adapted for this sourcebook.

Stages of Merkel Cell Carcinoma

After Merkel cell carcinoma has been diagnosed (found), more tests will be done to find out if cancer cells have spread from the place the cancer started to other parts of the body. The process used to find out whether the cancer has spread to other parts of the body is called staging. It is important to know the stage of the disease to plan the best treatment. The following stages are used for Merkel cell carcinoma:

Stage I

The primary tumor has not spread to lymph nodes or other parts of the body. Lymph nodes are small, bean-shaped structures that are found throughout the body. They produce and store infection-fighting cells.

Stage II

The cancer has spread to nearby lymph nodes, but has not spread to other parts of the body.

Stage III

The cancer has spread beyond nearby lymph nodes and to other parts of the body.

Recurrent Stage

Recurrent disease means that the cancer has recurred (come back) after it has been treated. It may come back in the same part of the body or in another part of the body.

How Is Merkel Cell Carcinoma Treated?

There are treatments for all patients with Merkel cell carcinoma. Three kinds of treatment are used:

- Surgery (taking out the cancer)

- Radiation therapy (using high-dose x-rays or other high-energy rays to kill cancer cells)
- Chemotherapy (using drugs to kill cancer cells)

Surgery

There are several different types of surgery that may be used to remove the tumor. These include:

- Wide surgical excision takes out the cancer and some of the skin around the tumor.
- Cryosurgery freezes the tumor and then removes it.
- Micrographic surgery is a tissue-sparing technique that removes only the tumor.

Radiation Therapy

Radiation therapy uses high-energy x-rays to kill cancer cells and shrink tumors. Radiation may come from a machine outside the body (external radiation therapy) or from putting materials that produce radiation (radioisotopes) through thin plastic tubes in the area where the cancer cells are found (internal radiation therapy).

Chemotherapy

Chemotherapy uses drugs to kill cancer cells. Chemotherapy may be taken by pill, or it may be put into the body by a needle in a vein or muscle. Chemotherapy is called a systemic treatment because the drugs enter the bloodstream, travel through the body, and can kill cancer cells throughout the body.

If a doctor removes all the cancer that can be seen at the time of the operation, a patient may be given chemotherapy after surgery to kill any cancer cells that are left. Chemotherapy given after an operation to a person who has no cancer cells that can be found is called adjuvant chemotherapy.

Treatment by Stage

Stage I Merkel Cell Carcinoma

Treatment may be one of the following:

1. Surgery alone.

2. Surgery followed by radiation therapy to the tumor site and regional lymph nodes.

Stage II Merkel Cell Carcinoma

Treatment may be one of the following:

1. Surgery alone.

2. Surgery followed by radiation therapy to the tumor site and regional lymph nodes.

3. Surgery with or without radiation therapy followed by adjuvant chemotherapy.

Stage III Merkel Cell Carcinoma

Treatment will probably be chemotherapy.

Recurrent Merkel Cell Carcinoma

Treatment may be one of the following:

1. Surgery alone.

2. Surgery followed by radiation therapy to the tumor site and regional lymph nodes.

3. Surgery with or without radiation therapy followed by adjuvant chemotherapy.

To Learn More

Call

For more information, U.S. residents may call the National Cancer Institute's (NCI's) Cancer Information Service toll-free at 1-800-4-CANCER (1-800-422-6237), Monday through Friday from 9:00 a.m. to 4:30 p.m. Deaf and hard-of-hearing callers with TTY equipment may call 1-800-332-8615. The call is free and a trained Cancer Information Specialist is available to answer your questions.

Web Sites and Organizations

The NCI's Cancer.gov Web site (**http://cancer.gov**) provides online access to information on cancer, clinical trials, and other Web sites and organizations that offer support and resources for cancer patients and their families. There are also many other places where people can get materials and information about cancer treatment and services. Local hospitals may have information on local and regional agencies that offer information about finances, getting to and from treatment, receiving care at home, and dealing with problems associated with cancer treatment.

Publications

The NCI has booklets and other materials for patients, health professionals, and the public. These publications discuss types of cancer, methods of cancer treatment, coping with cancer, and clinical trials. Some publications provide information on tests for cancer, cancer causes and prevention, cancer statistics, and NCI research activities. NCI materials on these and other topics may be ordered online or printed directly from the NCI Publications Locator (**https://cissecure.nci.nih.gov/ncipubs**). These materials can also be ordered by telephone from the Cancer Information Service toll-free at 1-800-4-CANCER (1-800-422-6237), TTY at 1-800-332-8615.

LiveHelp

The NCI's LiveHelp service, a program available on several of the Institute's Web sites, provides Internet users with the ability to chat online with an Information Specialist. The service is available from Monday - Friday 9:00

AM - 10:00 PM Eastern Time. Information Specialists can help Internet users find information on NCI Web sites and answer questions about cancer.

Write

For more information from the NCI, please write to this address:

National Cancer Institute
Office of Communications
31 Center Drive, MSC 2580
Bethesda, MD 20892-2580

About PDQ

PDQ Is a Comprehensive Cancer Database Available on Cancer.gov

PDQ is the National Cancer Institute's (NCI's) comprehensive cancer information database. Most of the information contained in PDQ is available online at Cancer.gov (**http://cancer.gov**), the NCI's Web site. PDQ is provided as a service of the NCI. The NCI is part of the National Institutes of Health, the federal government's focal point for biomedical research.

PDQ Contains Cancer Information Summaries

The PDQ database contains summaries of the latest published information on cancer prevention, detection, genetics, treatment, supportive care, and complementary and alternative medicine. Most summaries are available in two versions. The health professional versions provide detailed information written in technical language. The patient versions are written in easy-to-understand, non-technical language. Both versions provide current and accurate cancer information.

The PDQ cancer information summaries are developed by cancer experts and reviewed regularly. Editorial Boards made up of experts in oncology and related specialties are responsible for writing and maintaining the cancer information summaries. The summaries are reviewed regularly and changes are made as new information becomes available. The date on each summary ("Date Last Modified") indicates the time of the most recent change.

PDQ Contains Information on Clinical Trials

Before starting treatment, patients may want to think about taking part in a clinical trial. A clinical trial is a study to answer a scientific question, such as whether one treatment is better than another. Trials are based on past studies and what has been learned in the laboratory. Each trial answers certain scientific questions in order to find new and better ways to help cancer patients. During treatment clinical trials, information is collected about new treatments, the risks involved, and how well they do or do not work. If a clinical trial shows that a new treatment is better than one currently being used, the new treatment may become "standard."

Listings of clinical trials are included in PDQ and are available online at Cancer.gov (**http://cancer.gov/clinical_trials**). Descriptions of the trials are available in health professional and patient versions. Many cancer doctors who take part in clinical trials are also listed in PDQ. For more information, call the Cancer Information Service at 1-800-4-CANCER (1-800-422-6237); TTY at 1-800-332-8615.

More Guideline Sources

The guideline above on merkel cell carcinoma is only one example of the kind of material that you can find online and free of charge. The remainder of this chapter will direct you to other sources which either publish or can help you find additional guidelines on topics related to merkel cell carcinoma. Many of the guidelines listed below address topics that may be of particular relevance to your specific situation or of special interest to only some patients with merkel cell carcinoma. Due to space limitations these sources are listed in a concise manner. Do not hesitate to consult the following sources by either using the Internet hyperlink provided, or, in cases where the contact information is provided, contacting the publisher or author directly.

Topic Pages: MEDLINEplus

For patients wishing to go beyond guidelines published by specific Institutes of the NIH, the National Library of Medicine has created a vast and patient-oriented healthcare information portal called MEDLINEplus. Within this Internet-based system are "health topic pages." You can think of a health topic page as a guide to patient guides. To access this system, log on to **http://www.nlm.nih.gov/medlineplus/healthtopics.html**. From there you can either search using the alphabetical index or browse by broad topic areas. Recently, MEDLINEplus listed the following as being relevant to merkel cell carcinoma:

- Other Guides

    Basal cell carcinoma
    http://www.nlm.nih.gov/medlineplus/ency/article/000824.htm

    Squamous cell carcinoma
    http://www.nlm.nih.gov/medlineplus/ency/article/000829.htm

    Renal cell carcinoma
    http://www.nlm.nih.gov/medlineplus/ency/article/000516.htm

If you do not find topics of interest when browsing health topic pages, then you can choose to use the advanced search utility of MEDLINEplus at **http://www.nlm.nih.gov/medlineplus/advancedsearch.html**. This utility is similar to the NIH Search Utility, with the exception that it only includes material linked within the MEDLINEplus system (mostly patient-oriented information). It also has the disadvantage of generating unstructured results. We recommend, therefore, that you use this method only if you have a very targeted search.

The National Guideline Clearinghouse™

The National Guideline Clearinghouse™ offers hundreds of evidence-based clinical practice guidelines published in the United States and other countries. You can search their site located at **http://www.guideline.gov** by using the keyword "merkel cell carcinoma" or synonyms. The following was recently posted:

- **Procedure guideline for somatostatin receptor scintigraphy with In-111 pentetreotide.**

    Source: Society of Nuclear Medicine, Inc..; 2001 February 11; 9 pages

    http://www.guideline.gov/FRAMESETS/guideline_fs.asp?guideline=002176&sSearch_string=Merkel+cell+carcinoma

Healthfinder™

Healthfinder™ is an additional source sponsored by the U.S. Department of Health and Human Services which offers links to hundreds of other sites that contain healthcare information. This Web site is located at **http://www.healthfinder.gov**. Again, keyword searches can be used to find guidelines. The following was recently found in this database:

- **ABCD's of Skin Cancer**

    Summary: A general overview of three types of skin cancer-- basal cell carcinoma, squamous cell carcinoma, and melanoma are illustrated. Explains self-exam for skin cancer.

    Source: American Academy of Dermatology

    http://www.healthfinder.gov/scripts/recordpass.asp?RecordType=0&RecordID=5777

The NIH Search Utility

After browsing the references listed at the beginning of this chapter, you may want to explore the NIH Search Utility. This allows you to search for documents on over 100 selected Web sites that comprise the NIH-WEB-SPACE. Each of these servers is "crawled" and indexed on an ongoing basis. Your search will produce a list of various documents, all of which will relate in some way to merkel cell carcinoma. The drawbacks of this approach are that the information is not organized by theme and that the references are often a mix of information for professionals and patients. Nevertheless, a large number of the listed Web sites provide useful background information. We can only recommend this route, therefore, for relatively rare or specific disorders, or when using highly targeted searches. To use the NIH search utility, visit the following Web page: **http://search.nih.gov/index.html**.

Additional Web Sources

A number of Web sites that often link to government sites are available to the public. These can also point you in the direction of essential information. The following is a representative sample:

- AOL: **http://search.aol.com/cat.adp?id=168&layer=&from=subcats**
- drkoop.com®: **http://www.drkoop.com/conditions/ency/index.html**
- Family Village: **http://www.familyvillage.wisc.edu/specific.htm**
- Google: **http://directory.google.com/Top/Health/Conditions_and_Diseases/**
- Med Help International: **http://www.medhelp.org/HealthTopics/A.html**

- Open Directory Project:
  http://dmoz.org/Health/Conditions_and_Diseases/
- Yahoo.com: **http://dir.yahoo.com/Health/Diseases_and_Conditions/**
- WebMD®Health: **http://my.webmd.com/health_topics**

Vocabulary Builder

The material in this chapter may have contained a number of unfamiliar words. The following Vocabulary Builder introduces you to terms used in this chapter that have not been covered in the previous chapter:

Adjuvant: A substance which aids another, such as an auxiliary remedy; in immunology, nonspecific stimulator (e.g., BCG vaccine) of the immune response. [EU]

Aspiration: Removal of fluid from a lump, often a cyst, with a needle and a syringe. [NIH]

Basal cell carcinoma: A type of skin cancer that arises from the basal cells, small round cells found in the lower part (or base) of the epidermis, the outer layer of the skin. [NIH]

Biopsy: The removal of cells or tissues for examination under a microscope. When only a sample of tissue is removed, the procedure is called an incisional biopsy or core biopsy. When an entire tumor or lesion is removed, the procedure is called an excisional biopsy. When a sample of tissue or fluid is removed with a needle, the procedure is called a needle biopsy or fine-needle aspiration. [NIH]

Carcinoma: Cancer that begins in the skin or in tissues that line or cover internal organs. [NIH]

Cell: The individual unit that makes up all of the tissues of the body. All living things are made up of one or more cells. [NIH]

Chemotherapy: Treatment with anticancer drugs. [NIH]

Cryosurgery: Treatment performed with an instrument that freezes and destroys abnormal tissues. This procedure is a form of cryotherapy. [NIH]

Elasticity: Resistance and recovery from distortion of shape. [NIH]

Follicles: Shafts through which hair grows. [NIH]

Implantation: The insertion or grafting into the body of biological, living, inert, or radioactive material. [EU]

Invasive: 1. having the quality of invasiveness. 2. involving puncture or incision of the skin or insertion of an instrument or foreign material into the body; said of diagnostic techniques. [EU]

Liver: A large, glandular organ located in the upper abdomen. The liver cleanses the blood and aids in digestion by secreting bile. [NIH]

Lymph: The almost colorless fluid that travels through the lymphatic system and carries cells that help fight infection and disease. [NIH]

Malignant: Cancerous; a growth with a tendency to invade and destroy nearby tissue and spread to other parts of the body. [NIH]

Melanoma: A form of skin cancer that arises in melanocytes, the cells that produce pigment. Melanoma usually begins in a mole. [NIH]

Metastasize: To spread from one part of the body to another. When cancer cells metastasize and form secondary tumors, the cells in the metastatic tumor are like those in the original (primary) tumor. [NIH]

Molecular: Of, pertaining to, or composed of molecules : a very small mass of matter. [EU]

Neuroendocrine: Having to do with the interactions between the nervous system and the endocrine system. Describes certain cells that release hormones into the blood in response to stimulation of the nervous system. [NIH]

Oncology: The study of cancer. [NIH]

Radioisotope: An unstable element that releases radiation as it breaks down. Radioisotopes can be used in imaging tests or as a treatment for cancer. [NIH]

Receptor: A molecule inside or on the surface of a cell that binds to a specific substance and causes a specific physiologic effect in the cell. [NIH]

Somatostatin: A polypeptide hormone produced in the hypothalamus, and other tissues and organs. It inhibits the release of human growth hormone, and also modulates important physiological functions of the kidney, pancreas, and gastrointestinal tract. Somatostatin receptors are widely expressed throughout the body. Somatostatin also acts as a neurotransmitter in the central and peripheral nervous systems. [NIH]

Species: A taxonomic category subordinate to a genus (or subgenus) and superior to a subspecies or variety, composed of individuals possessing common characters distinguishing them from other categories of individuals of the same taxonomic level. In taxonomic nomenclature, species are designated by the genus name followed by a Latin or Latinized adjective or noun. [EU]

Squamous cell carcinoma: Cancer that begins in squamous cells, which are thin, flat cells resembling fish scales. Squamous cells are found in the tissue that forms the surface of the skin, the lining of the hollow organs of the body, and the passages of the respiratory and digestive tracts. Also called epidermoid carcinoma. [NIH]

Staging: Performing exams and tests to learn the extent of the cancer within the body, especially whether the disease has spread from the original site to other parts of the body. [NIH]

Systemic: Affecting the entire body. [NIH]

Thoracic: Having to do with the chest. [NIH]

Transfusion: The infusion of components of blood or whole blood into the bloodstream. The blood may be donated from another person, or it may have been taken from the person earlier and stored until needed. [NIH]

CHAPTER 2. SEEKING GUIDANCE

Overview

Some patients are comforted by the knowledge that a number of organizations dedicate their resources to helping people with merkel cell carcinoma. These associations can become invaluable sources of information and advice. Many associations offer aftercare support, financial assistance, and other important services. Furthermore, healthcare research has shown that support groups often help people to better cope with their conditions.[7] In addition to support groups, your physician can be a valuable source of guidance and support. Therefore, finding a physician that can work with your unique situation is a very important aspect of your care.

In this chapter, we direct you to resources that can help you find patient organizations and medical specialists. We begin by describing how to find associations and peer groups that can help you better understand and cope with merkel cell carcinoma. The chapter ends with a discussion on how to find a doctor that is right for you.

Associations and Merkel Cell Carcinoma

As mentioned by the Agency for Healthcare Research and Quality, sometimes the emotional side of an illness can be as taxing as the physical side.[8] You may have fears or feel overwhelmed by your situation. Everyone has different ways of dealing with disease or physical injury. Your attitude, your expectations, and how well you cope with your condition can all

---

[7] Churches, synagogues, and other houses of worship might also have groups that can offer you the social support you need.
[8] This section has been adapted from **http://www.ahcpr.gov/consumer/diaginf5.htm**.

influence your well-being. This is true for both minor conditions and serious illnesses. For example, a study on female breast cancer survivors revealed that women who participated in support groups lived longer and experienced better quality of life when compared with women who did not participate. In the support group, women learned coping skills and had the opportunity to share their feelings with other women in the same situation.

In addition to associations or groups that your doctor might recommend, we suggest that you consider the following list (if there is a fee for an association, you may want to check with your insurance provider to find out if the cost will be covered):

- **American Skin Association**

    Address: American Skin Association 150 East 58th Street, 33rd Floor, New York, NY 10155-0002

    Telephone: (212) 753-8260 Toll-free: (800) 499-7546

    Fax: (212) 688-6547

    Email: AmericanSkin@compuserve.com

    Web Site: None

    Background: The American Skin Association (ASA) is a national nonprofit organization dedicated to building a network of lay people to achieve more effective prevention, treatment, and cure of skin disorders. ASA programs include generating support for skin research and providing information and education to the public regarding the skin and its disorders. ASA's mission is to identify, promote, and support research in biology of the skin, stimulate the transfer of advances in the field to clinical care of dermatology patients, and educate the community regarding diseases, symptoms, and care of the skin. To meet this goal, the Association engages in fundraising to support research and develops local chapters throughout the country. Information on a wide spectrum of skin disorders is available including 'Your Newborn's Skin and the Sun,' 'Ultraviolet Index: What You Need To Know,' 'Outdoor Sports and Your Skin,' and 'Proper Skin Care Can Make Gardening a Bed of Roses.' Founded in 1987, ASA also publishes 'SkinFacts,' a quarterly newsletter.

    Relevant area(s) of interest: Melanoma, Skin Cancer

- **CancerOnline**

    Address:

    Telephone: (212) 753-8260 Toll-free: (800) 499-7546

    Email: cancerinfo@stonecottage.com

Web Site: http://www.canceronline.org

Background: CancerOnline is a nonprofit site on the Internet dedicated to providing individuals with cancer easy access to clinical information and offering extensive practical support and encouragement. CancerOnline collaborates with many different cancer care centers and organizations and provides original material contributed by cancer patients, caregivers, and cancer care specialists in private practice and a variety of cancer centers. CancerOnline's content is overseen by three advisory panels made up of oncologists, radiologists, and clinical care providers who want to help cancer patients become students of their disease; other cancer care specialists and providers of psychosocial support who want to encourage patients to participate actively in their treatment; and patients, survivors, and caregivers who want to help patients live with vitality and hope even in the face of a life-challenging illness. CancerOnline offers several major areas within its site including 'About CancerOnline,' 'Support and Encouragement,' 'Getting Information,' 'Participating in This Community,' and 'Special Features.' The site offers several sources of clinical information that can be accessed through a network of subject areas; practical advice before, during, and after treatment; stories from individuals who have triumphed over cancer; opportunities for affected individuals and families to contribute personal stories, creative expressions, commentaries, and questions; hints on how to obtain additional information on and off the Internet; dynamic linkage to additional web sites that provide information and support to those with particular types of cancer; and more. CancerOnline provides information and support to individuals with any type of cancer including Bladder Cancer, Breast Cancer, Colon and Rectal Cancer, Liver Cancer, Lymphoma, Ovarian Cancer, Prostate Cancer, Stomach Cancer, Uterine Cancer, Pediatric Cancers, Brain Tumors, Head and Neck Cancer, Leukemia, Lung Cancer, Melanoma, Pancreatic Cancer, Skin Cancer, Thyroid Cancer, and Rare Adult Cancers.

Relevant area(s) of interest: Melanoma

- **International Cancer Alliance for Research and Education**

   Address: International Cancer Alliance for Research and Education 4853 Cordell Avenue, Suite 11, Bethesda, MD 20814

   Telephone: (301) 654-7933 Toll-free: (800) 422-7361

   Fax: (301) 654-8684

   Email: info@icare.org

   Web Site: http://icare.org

Background: The International Cancer Alliance for Research and Education (ICARE) is a nonprofit organization that provides focused information to individuals affected by cancer and their physicians on an ongoing, person-to-person basis. Cancer is a general term referring to a group of diseases characterized by uncontrolled cellular growth that may invade surrounding tissues and spread (metastasize) to other bodily tissues or organs. The different cancers may be classified based upon the organ and cell type involved, the nature of the malignancy, and the disease's clinical course. ICARE has developed several patient-centered programs through a process of collection, evaluation, and dissemination of information, bringing affected individuals into contact with physicians and scientists from around the world. The Alliance is operated by a network of scientists, clinicians, staff members, and lay volunteers, many of whom are affected by cancer themselves. The Alliance maintains the ICARE Registry, a confidential membership listing that permits ongoing dialogue between ICARE and its network members. Registry members receive a 'cancer therapy review' including a description of the specific form of cancer in question, information concerning detection and staging procedures, an overview of current treatments, a bibliography for more in-depth research, and listings of diagnostic tests, ongoing clinical trials, and second opinion centers. Registry members also receive medical, research, clinical trial, and Food and Drug Administration (FDA) updates relating to the specific form of cancer or cancer in general; regular newsletters; and access to all ICARE programs. Such programs include ICARE patient education partner centers, which provide affected individuals with access to an electronic library of cancer information and online hook-ups at the community level; private electronic support groups for individuals dealing with common types of cancer or common issues; a clinical trial matching program; and other services. ICARE provides information concerning its mission, objectives, services, and programs on its web site on the Internet.

Relevant area(s) of interest: Melanoma

- **Nevus Outreach, Inc**

    Address: Nevus Outreach, Inc. 1616 Alpha Street, Lansing, MI 48910

    Telephone: (517) 487-2306

    Fax: (517) 374-7610

    Email: info@nevus.org

    Web Site: http://www.nevus.org

    Background: Nevus Outreach, Inc. (NOI) is a voluntary health organization formed in 1997 by a group of parents dedicated to improving medical knowledge and treatment for individuals with giant congenital nevi and related disorders such as neurocutaneous melanosis. Giant congenital nevi are large, darkly pigmented moles or birthmarks (nevi) that are present at birth (congenital). Although such nevi may vary in size and shape and may cover any area of the body, they are often present on the chest, the shoulders, the upper back, the area covered by bathing trunks, the lower arms and legs, and/or various areas on the face and/or scalp. Individuals with giant nevi have an abnormally increased risk of developing malignant melanoma, a form of skin cancer. In addition, the nevus cells that appear on the skin may form in the central nervous system (neurocutaneous melanosis), which may cause neurological abnormalities and potentially life-threatening complications. The Nevus Outreach is committed to providing information, assistance, and support to affected individuals and family members; promoting additional research; and increasing awareness of these conditions among dermatologists and other health care professionals. NOI provides understandable information on these disorders; publishes a biannual newsletter entitled 'Nevus News'; provides periodic updates on important events and announcements; and sponsors an annual conference to enable affected individuals and family members to network with one another and to interact with medical specialists in the field. The Nevus Outreach also acts as an advocate for affected families, helps make travel assistance arrangements for treatment, and provides referrals to other relevant organizations. In addition, the NOI has a Web site on the Internet that provides information on nevi disorders, online networking opportunities, and dynamic links to other helpful sources of information and support.

- **Skin Cancer Foundation**

  Address: Skin Cancer Foundation 245 Fifth Avenue, Suite 1403, New York, NY 10016

  Telephone: (212) 725-5176 Toll-free: (800) 754-6490

  Fax: (212) 725-5751

  Email: info@skincancer.org

  Background: The Skin Cancer Foundation is a not-for-profit international educational health organization dedicated to providing information on detection and prevention of and support to individuals with skin cancer. The Foundation seeks to educate the public about the different forms of skin cancer and promotes and supports ongoing medical research into the causes and treatment of these diseases. Established in 1977, the Skin Cancer Foundation has a growing membership of over 130 leading physicians. The Foundation provides support for medical research and training; functions as a major resource center for the media; and works to educate the public. Programs include screening clinics, health fairs, and corporate and community wellness programs. Educational materials produced by the organization include a wide variety of brochures, posters, books, newsletters, and audio-visual materials.

Relevant area(s) of interest: Melanoma, Skin Cancer

Finding More Associations

There are a number of directories that list additional medical associations that you may find useful. While not all of these directories will provide different information than what is listed above, by consulting all of them, you will have nearly exhausted all sources for patient associations.

The National Cancer Institute (NCI)

The National Cancer Institute (NCI) has complied a list of national organizations that offer services to people with cancer and their families. To view the list, see the NCI fact sheet online at the following Web address: **http://cis.nci.nih.gov/fact/8_1.htm**. The name of each organization is accompanied by its contact information and a brief explanation of its services.

The National Health Information Center (NHIC)

The National Health Information Center (NHIC) offers a free referral service to help people find organizations that provide information about merkel cell carcinoma. For more information, see the NHIC's Web site at **http://www.health.gov/NHIC/** or contact an information specialist by calling 1-800-336-4797.

DIRLINE

A comprehensive source of information on associations is the DIRLINE database maintained by the National Library of Medicine. The database comprises some 10,000 records of organizations, research centers, and government institutes and associations which primarily focus on health and biomedicine. DIRLINE is available via the Internet at the following Web site: **http://dirline.nlm.nih.gov/**. Simply type in "merkel cell carcinoma" (or a synonym) or the name of a topic, and the site will list information contained in the database on all relevant organizations.

The Combined Health Information Database

Another comprehensive source of information on healthcare associations is the Combined Health Information Database. Using the "Detailed Search" option, you will need to limit your search to "Organizations" and "merkel cell carcinoma". Type the following hyperlink into your Web browser: **http://chid.nih.gov/detail/detail.html**. To find associations, use the drop boxes at the bottom of the search page where "You may refine your search by." For publication date, select "All Years." Then, select your preferred language and the format option "Organization Resource Sheet." By making these selections and typing in "merkel cell carcinoma" (or synonyms) into the "For these words:" box, you will only receive results on organizations dealing with merkel cell carcinoma. You should check back periodically with this database since it is updated every 3 months.

The National Organization for Rare Disorders, Inc.

The National Organization for Rare Disorders, Inc. has prepared a Web site that provides, at no charge, lists of associations organized by specific diseases. You can access this database at the following Web site: **http://www.rarediseases.org/cgi-bin/nord/searchpage**. Select the option called "Organizational Database (ODB)" and type "merkel cell carcinoma" (or a synonym) in the search box.

Cancer Support Groups[9]

People diagnosed with cancer and their families face many challenges that may leave them feeling overwhelmed, afraid, and alone. It can be difficult to cope with these challenges or to talk to even the most supportive family members and friends. Often, support groups can help people affected by cancer feel less alone and can improve their ability to deal with the uncertainties and challenges that cancer brings. Support groups give people

---

[9] This section has been adapted from the NCI: **http://cis.nci.nih.gov/fact/8_8.htm**.

who are affected by similar diseases an opportunity to meet and discuss ways to cope with the illness.

How Can Support Groups Help?

People who have been diagnosed with cancer sometimes find they need assistance coping with the emotional as well as the practical aspects of their disease. In fact, attention to the emotional burden of cancer is sometimes part of a patient's treatment plan. Cancer support groups are designed to provide a confidential atmosphere where cancer patients or cancer survivors can discuss the challenges that accompany the illness with others who may have experienced the same challenges. For example, people gather to discuss the emotional needs created by cancer, to exchange information about their disease—including practical problems such as managing side effects or returning to work after treatment—and to share their feelings. Support groups have helped thousands of people cope with these and similar situations.

Can Family Members and Friends Participate in Support Groups?

Family and friends are affected when cancer touches someone they love, and they may need help in dealing with stresses such as family disruptions, financial worries, and changing roles within relationships. To help meet these needs, some support groups are designed just for family members of people diagnosed with cancer; other groups encourage families and friends to participate along with the cancer patient or cancer survivor.

How Can People Find Support Groups?

Many organizations offer support groups for people diagnosed with cancer and their family members or friends. The NCI fact sheet *National Organizations That Offer Services to People with Cancer and Their Families* lists many cancer-concerned organizations that can provide information about support groups. This fact sheet is available at **http://cis.nci.nih.gov/fact/8_1.htm** on the Internet, or can be ordered from the Cancer Information Service at 1–800–4–CANCER (1–800–422–6237). Some of these organizations provide information on their Web sites about contacting support groups.

Doctors, nurses, or hospital social workers who work with cancer patients may also have information about support groups, such as their location, size, type, and how often they meet. Most hospitals have social services departments that provide information about cancer support programs. Additionally, many newspapers carry a special health supplement containing information about where to find support groups.

What Types of Support Groups Are Available?

Several kinds of support groups are available to meet the individual needs of people at all stages of cancer treatment, from diagnosis through follow-up care. Some groups are general cancer support groups, while more specialized groups may be for teens or young adults, for family members, or for people affected by a particular disease. Support groups may be led by a professional, such as a psychiatrist, psychologist, or social worker, or by cancer patients or survivors. In addition, support groups can vary in approach, size, and how often they meet. Many groups are free, but some require a fee (people can contact their health insurance company to find out whether their plan will cover the cost). It is important for people to find an atmosphere that is comfortable and meets their individual needs.

Online Support Groups

In addition to support groups, commercial Internet service providers offer forums and chat rooms for people with different illnesses and conditions. WebMD®, for example, offers such a service at their Web site: **http://boards.webmd.com/roundtable**. These online self-help communities can help you connect with a network of people whose concerns are similar to yours. Online support groups are places where people can talk informally. If you read about a novel approach, consult with your doctor or other healthcare providers, as the treatments or discoveries you hear about may not be scientifically proven to be safe and effective.

The Cancer Information Service[10]

The Cancer Information Service (CIS) is a program of the National Cancer Institute (NCI), the Nation's lead agency for cancer research. As a resource for information and education about cancer, the CIS is a leader in helping

---

[10] This section has been adapted from the NCI: **http://cis.nci.nih.gov/fact/2_5.htm**.

people become active participants in their own health care by providing the latest information on cancer in understandable language. Through its network of regional offices, the CIS serves the United States, Puerto Rico, the U.S. Virgin Islands, and the Pacific Islands.

For 25 years, the Cancer Information Service has provided the latest and most accurate cancer information to patients and families, the public, and health professionals by:

- Interacting with people one-on-one through its Information Service,
- Working with organizations through its Partnership Program,
- Participating in research efforts to find the best ways to help people adopt healthier behaviors,
- Providing access to NCI information over the Internet.

How Does the CIS Assist the Public?

Through the CIS toll-free telephone service (1-800-4-CANCER), callers speak with knowledgeable, caring staff who are experienced at explaining medical information in easy-to-understand terms. CIS information specialists answer calls in English and Spanish. They also provide cancer information to deaf and hard of hearing callers through the toll-free TTY number (1-800-332-8615). CIS staff have access to comprehensive, accurate information from the NCI on a range of cancer topics, including the most recent advances in cancer treatment. They take as much time as each caller needs, provide thorough and personalized attention, and keep all calls confidential.

The CIS also provides live, online assistance to users of NCI Web sites through LiveHelp, an instant messaging service that is available from 9:00 a.m. to 7:30 p.m. Eastern time, Monday through Friday. Through LiveHelp, information specialists provide answers to questions about cancer and help in navigating Cancer.gov, the NCI's Web site.

Through the telephone numbers or LiveHelp service, CIS users receive:

- Answers to their questions about cancer, including ways to prevent cancer, symptoms and risks, diagnosis, current treatments, and research studies;
- Written materials from the NCI;
- Referrals to clinical trials and cancer-related services, such as treatment centers, mammography facilities, or other cancer organizations;

- Assistance in quitting smoking from information specialists trained in smoking cessation counseling.

What Kind of Assistance Does the CIS Partnership Program Offer?

Through its Partnership Program, the CIS collaborates with established national, state, and regional organizations to reach minority and medically underserved audiences with cancer information. Partnership Program staff provide assistance to organizations developing programs that focus on breast and cervical cancer, clinical trials, tobacco control, and cancer awareness for special populations. To reach those in need, the CIS:

- Helps bring cancer information to people who do not traditionally seek health information or who may have difficulties doing so because of educational, financial, cultural, or language barriers;

- Provides expertise to organizations to help strengthen their ability to inform people they serve about cancer; and

- Links organizations with similar goals and helps them plan and evaluate programs, develop coalitions, conduct training on cancer-related topics, and use NCI resources.

How Do CIS Research Efforts Assist the Public?

The CIS plays an important role in research by studying the most effective ways to communicate with people about healthy lifestyles; health risks; and options for preventing, diagnosing, and treating cancer. The ability to conduct health communications research is a unique aspect of the CIS. Results from these research studies can be applied to improving the way the CIS communicates about cancer and can help other programs communicate more effectively.

How Do People Reach the Cancer Information Service?

- To speak with a CIS information specialist call 1-800-4-CANCER (1-800-422-6237), 9:00 a.m. to 4:30 p.m. local time, Monday through Friday. Deaf or hard of hearing callers with TTY equipment may call 1-800-332-8615.

- To obtain online assistance visit the NCI's Cancer Information Web site at **http://cancer.gov/cancer_information** and click on the LiveHelp link between 9:00 a.m. and 7:30 p.m. Eastern time, Monday through Friday.

- For information 24 hours a day, 7 days a week call 1-800-4-CANCER and select option 4 to hear recorded information at any time.
- Visit NCI's Web site at **http://cancer.gov** on the Internet.
- Visit the CIS Web site at **http://cancer.gov/cis** on the Internet.

Finding Cancer Resources in Your Community[11]

If you have cancer or are undergoing cancer treatment, there are places in your community to turn to for help. There are many local organizations throughout the country that offer a variety of practical and support services to people with cancer. However, people often don't know about these services or are unable to find them. National cancer organizations can assist you in finding these resources, and there are a number of things you can do for yourself.

Whether you are looking for a support group, counseling, advice, financial assistance, transportation to and from treatment, or information about cancer, most neighborhood organizations, local health care providers, or area hospitals are a good place to start. Often, the hardest part of looking for help is knowing the right questions to ask.

What Kind of Help Can I Get?

Until now, you probably never thought about the many issues and difficulties that arise with a diagnosis of cancer. There are support services to help you deal with almost any type of problem that might occur. The first step in finding the help you need is knowing what types of services are available. The following pages describe some of these services and how to find them.

- **Information on Cancer.** Most national cancer organizations provide a range of information services, including materials on different types of cancer, treatments, and treatment-related issues.
- **Counseling.** While some people are reluctant to seek counseling, studies show that having someone to talk to reduces stress and helps people both mentally and physically. Counseling can also provide emotional support to cancer patients and help them better understand their illness. Different types of counseling include individual, group, family, self-help

---

[11] Adapted from the NCI: **http://cis.nci.nih.gov/fact/8_9.htm**.

(sometimes called peer counseling), bereavement, patient-to-patient, and sexuality.

- **Medical Treatment Decisions.** Often, people with cancer need to make complicated medical decisions. Many organizations provide hospital and physician referrals for second opinions and information on clinical trials (research studies with people), which may expand treatment options.

- **Prevention and Early Detection.** While cancer prevention may never be 100 percent effective, many things (such as quitting smoking and eating healthy foods) can greatly reduce a person's risk for developing cancer. Prevention services usually focus on smoking cessation and nutrition. Early detection services, which are designed to detect cancer when a person has no symptoms of disease, can include referrals for screening mammograms, Pap tests, or prostate exams.

- **Home Health Care.** Home health care assists patients who no longer need to stay in a hospital or nursing home, but still require professional medical help. Skilled nursing care, physical therapy, social work services, and nutrition counseling are all available at home.

- **Hospice Care.** Hospice is care focused on the special needs of terminally ill cancer patients. Sometimes called *palliative care*, it centers around providing comfort, controlling physical symptoms, and giving emotional support to patients who can no longer benefit from curative treatment. Hospice programs provide services in various settings, including the patient's home, hospice centers, hospitals, or skilled nursing facilities. Your doctor or social worker can provide a referral for these services.

- **Rehabilitation.** Rehabilitation services help people adjust to the effects of cancer and its treatment. Physical rehabilitation focuses on recovery from the physical effects of surgery or the side effects associated with chemotherapy. Occupational or vocational therapy helps people readjust to everyday routines, get back to work, or find employment.

- **Advocacy.** Advocacy is a general term that refers to promoting or protecting the rights and interests of a certain group, such as cancer patients. Advocacy groups may offer services to assist with legal, ethical, medical, employment, legislative, or insurance issues, among others. For instance, if you feel your insurance company has not handled your claim fairly, you may want to advocate for a review of its decision.

- **Financial.** Having cancer can be a tremendous financial burden to cancer patients and their families. There are programs sponsored by the government and nonprofit organizations to help cancer patients with problems related to medical billing, insurance coverage, and reimbursement issues. There are also sources for financial assistance, and ways to get help collecting entitlements from Medicaid, Medicare, and the Social Security Administration.

- **Housing/Lodging.** Some organizations provide lodging for the family of a patient undergoing treatment, especially if it is a child who is ill and the parents are required to accompany the child to treatment.
- **Children's Services.** A number of organizations provide services for children with cancer, including summer camps, make-a-wish programs, and help for parents seeking child care.

How to Find These Services

Often, the services that people with cancer are looking for are right in their own neighborhood or city. The following is a list of places where you can begin your search for help.

- The hospital, clinic, or medical center where you see your doctor, received your diagnosis, or where you undergo treatment should be able to give you information. Your doctor or nurse may be able to tell you about your specific medical condition, pain management, rehabilitation services, home nursing, or hospice care.
- Most hospitals also have a social work, home care, or discharge planning department. This department may be able to help you find a support group, a nonprofit agency that helps people who have cancer, or the government agencies that oversee Social Security, Medicare, and Medicaid. While you are undergoing treatment, be sure to ask the hospital about transportation, practical assistance, or even temporary child care. Talk to a hospital financial counselor in the business office about developing a monthly payment plan if you need help with hospital expenses.
- The public library is an excellent source of information, as are patient libraries at many cancer centers. A librarian can help you find books and articles through a literature search.
- A local church, synagogue, YMCA or YWCA, or fraternal order may provide financial assistance, or may have volunteers who can help with transportation and home care. Catholic Charities, the United Way, or the American Red Cross may also operate local offices. Some of these organizations may provide home care, and the United Way's information and referral service can refer you to an agency that provides financial help. To find the United Way serving your community, visit their online

directory at **http://www.unitedway.org** on the Internet or look in the White Pages of your local telephone book.

- Local or county government agencies may offer low-cost transportation (sometimes called para-transit) to individuals unable to use public transportation. Most states also have an Area Agency on Aging that offers low-cost services to people over 60. Your hospital or community social worker can direct you to government agencies for entitlements, including Social Security, state disability, Medicaid, income maintenance, and food stamps. (Keep in mind that most applications to entitlement programs take some time to process.) The Federal government also runs the Hill-Burton program (1-800-638-0742), which funds certain medical facilities and hospitals to provide cancer patients with free or low-cost care if they are in financial need.

Getting the Most From a Service: What To Ask

No matter what type of help you are looking for, the only way to find resources to fit your needs is to ask the right questions. When you are calling an organization for information, it is important to think about what questions you are going to ask before you call. Many people find it helpful to write out their questions in advance, and to take notes during the call. Another good tip is to ask the name of the person with whom you are speaking in case you have follow-up questions. Below are some of the questions you may want to consider if you are calling or visiting a new agency and want to learn about how they can help:

- How do I apply [for this service]?
- Are there eligibility requirements? What are they?
- Is there an application process? How long will it take? What information will I need to complete the application process? Will I need anything else to get the service?
- Do you have any other suggestions or ideas about where I can find help?

The most important thing to remember is that you will rarely receive help unless you ask for it. In fact, asking can be the hardest part of getting help. Don't be afraid or ashamed to ask for assistance. Cancer is a very difficult disease, but there are people and services that can ease your burdens and help you focus on your treatment and recovery.

Finding Doctors Who Specialize in Cancer Care[12]

One of the most important aspects of your treatment will be the relationship between you and your doctor or specialist. All patients with merkel cell carcinoma must go through the process of selecting a physician. A common way to find a doctor who specializes in cancer care is to ask for a referral from your primary care physician. Sometimes, you may know a specialist yourself, or through the experience of a family member, coworker, or friend.

The following resources may also be able to provide you with names of doctors who specialize in treating specific diseases or conditions. However, these resources may not have information about the quality of care that the doctors provide.

- Your local hospital or its patient referral service may be able to provide you with a list of specialists who practice at that hospital.

- Your nearest National Cancer Institute (NCI)-designated cancer center can provide information about doctors who practice at that center. The NCI fact sheet *The National Cancer Institute Cancer Centers Program* describes and gives contact information, including Web sites, for NCI-designated cancer treatment centers around the country. Many of the cancer centers' Web sites have searchable directories of physicians who practice at each facility. The NCI's fact sheet is available at **http://cis.nci.nih.gov/fact/1_2.htm** on the Internet, or by calling the Cancer Information Service (CIS) at 1-800-4-CANCER (1-800-422-6237).

- The American Board of Medical Specialties (ABMS) publishes a list of board-certified physicians. The *Official ABMS Directory of Board Certified Medical Specialists* lists doctors' names along with their specialty and their educational background. This resource is available in most public libraries. The ABMS also has a Web site that can be used to verify whether a specific physician is board-certified. This free service is located at **http://www.abms.org/newsearch.asp** on the Internet. Verification of a physician's board certification can also be obtained by calling the ABMS at 1-866-275-2267 (1-866-ASK-ABMS).

- The American Medical Association (AMA) provides an online service called AMA Physician Select that offers basic professional information on virtually every licensed physician in the United States and its possessions. The database can be searched by doctor's name or by medical specialty. The AMA Physician Select service is located at **http://www.ama-assn.org/aps/amahg.htm** on the Internet.

---

[12] Adapted from the NCI: **http://cis.nci.nih.gov/fact/7_47.htm**.

- The American Society of Clinical Oncologists (ASCO) provides an online list of doctors who are members of ASCO. The member database has the names and affiliations of over 15,000 oncologists worldwide. It can be searched by doctor's name, institution's name, location, and/or type of board certification. This service is located at **http://www.asco.org/people/db/html/m_db.htm** on the Internet.

- The American College of Surgeons (ACOS) Fellowship Database is an online list of surgeons who are Fellows of the ACOS. The list can be searched by doctor's name, geographic location, or medical specialty. This service is located at **http://web.facs.org/acsdir/default.htm** on the Internet. The ACOS can be contacted at 633 North Saint Clair Street, Chicago, IL 60611-3211; or by telephone at 312-202-5000.

- Local medical societies may maintain lists of doctors in each specialty.

- Public and medical libraries may have print directories of doctors' names, listed geographically by specialty.

- Your local Yellow Pages may have doctors listed by specialty under "Physicians."

The Agency for Healthcare Research and Quality (AHRQ) offers *Your Guide to Choosing Quality Health Care*, which has information for consumers on choosing a health plan, a doctor, a hospital, or a long-term care provider. The Guide includes suggestions and checklists that you can use to determine which doctor or hospital is best for you. This resource is available at **http://www.ahrq.gov/consumer/qntool.htm** on the Internet. You can also order the Guide by calling the AHRQ Publications Clearinghouse at 1-800-358-9295.

If you are a member of a health insurance plan, your choice may be limited to doctors who participate in your plan. Your insurance company can provide you with a list of participating primary care doctors and specialists. It is important to ask your insurance company if the doctor you choose is accepting new patients through your health plan. You also have the option of seeing a doctor outside your health plan and paying the costs yourself. If you have a choice of health insurance plans, you may first wish to consider which doctor or doctors you would like to use, then choose a plan that includes your chosen physician(s).

The National Comprehensive Cancer Network (NCCN) Physician Directory lists specialists who practice in the NCCN's 19 member institutions across the U.S. To access the directory, go to **http://www.nccn.org/** and click on "Physician Directory". To use this service, you will be required to scroll to the bottom of the page and select "I agree." Enter your search criteria and select "Find" at the bottom of the page. To obtain more information on a physician or institution, contact the institution's Physician Referral Department or the NCCN Patient Information and Referral Service at 1-888-909-NCCN or **patientinformation@nccn.org**.

If the previous sources did not meet your needs, you may want to log on to the Web site of the National Organization for Rare Disorders (NORD) at **http://www.rarediseases.org/**. NORD maintains a database of doctors with expertise in various rare diseases. The Metabolic Information Network (MIN), 800-945-2188, also maintains a database of physicians with expertise in various metabolic diseases.

Selecting Your Doctor[3]

There are many factors to consider when choosing a doctor. To make the most informed decision, you may wish to speak with several doctors before choosing one. When you meet with each doctor, you might want to consider the following:

- Does the doctor have the education and training to meet my needs?
- Does the doctor use the hospital that I have chosen?
- Does the doctor listen to me and treat me with respect?
- Does the doctor explain things clearly and encourage me to ask questions?
- What are the doctor's office hours?
- Who covers for the doctor when he or she is unavailable? Will that person have access to my medical records?
- How long does it take to get an appointment with the doctor?

If you are choosing a surgeon, you may wish to ask additional questions about the surgeon's background and experience with specific procedures. These questions may include:

- Is the surgeon board-certified?[14]

---

[13] This section has been adapted from the AHRQ: **http://www.ahrq.gov/consumer/qntascii/qntdr.htm**
[14] While board certification is a good measure of a doctor's knowledge, it is possible to receive quality care from doctors who are not board certified.

- Has the surgeon been evaluated by a national professional association of surgeons, such as the American College of Surgeons (ACOS)?
- At which treatment facility or facilities does the surgeon practice?
- How often does the surgeon perform the type of surgery I need?
- How many of these procedures has the surgeon performed? What was the success rate?

It is important for you to feel comfortable with the specialist that you choose, because you will be working closely with that person to make decisions about your cancer treatment. Trust your own observations and feelings when deciding on a doctor for your medical care.

Other health professionals and support services may also be important during cancer treatment. The National Cancer Institute fact sheet *Your Health Care Team: Your Doctor Is Only the Beginning* has information about these providers and services, and how to locate them. This fact sheet is located at **http://cis.nci.nih.gov/fact/8_10.htm** on the Internet, or can be obtained by calling the CIS at 1-800-4-CANCER (1-800-422-6237).

Working with Your Doctor[15]

Research has shown that patients who have good relationships with their doctors tend to be more satisfied with their care and have better results. Here are some tips to help you and your doctor become partners:

- You know important things about your symptoms and your health history. Tell your doctor what you think he or she needs to know.
- It is important to tell your doctor personal information, even if it makes you feel embarrassed or uncomfortable.
- Bring a "health history" list with you (and keep it up to date).
- Always bring any medications you are currently taking with you to the appointment, or you can bring a list of your medications including dosage and frequency information. Talk about any allergies or reactions you have had to your medications.
- Tell your doctor about any natural or alternative medicines you are taking.

---

[15] This section has been adapted from the AHRQ: **www.ahrq.gov/consumer/qntascii/qntdr.htm**.

- Bring other medical information, such as x-ray films, test results, and medical records.
- Ask questions. If you don't, your doctor will assume that you understood everything that was said.
- Write down your questions before your visit. List the most important ones first to make sure that they are addressed.
- Consider bringing a friend with you to the appointment to help you ask questions. This person can also help you understand and/or remember the answers.
- Ask your doctor to draw pictures if you think that this would help you understand.
- Take notes. Some doctors do not mind if you bring a tape recorder to help you remember things, but always ask first.
- Let your doctor know if you need more time. If there is not time that day, perhaps you can speak to a nurse or physician assistant on staff or schedule a telephone appointment.
- Take information home. Ask for written instructions. Your doctor may also have brochures and audio and videotapes that can help you.
- After leaving the doctor's office, take responsibility for your care. If you have questions, call. If your symptoms get worse or if you have problems with your medication, call. If you had tests and do not hear from your doctor, call for your test results. If your doctor recommended that you have certain tests, schedule an appointment to get them done. If your doctor said you should see an additional specialist, make an appointment.

By following these steps, you will enhance the relationship you will have with your physician.

Finding a Cancer Treatment Facility[16]

Choosing a treatment facility is another important consideration for getting the best medical care possible. Although you may not be able to choose which hospital treats you in an emergency, you can choose a facility for scheduled and ongoing care. If you have already found a doctor for your cancer treatment, you may need to choose a facility based on where your

---

[16] Adapted from the NCI: **http://cis.nci.nih.gov/fact/7_47.htm**. At this Web site, information on how to find treatment facilities is also available for patients living outside the U.S.

doctor practices. Your doctor may be able to recommend a facility that provides quality care to meet your needs. You may wish to ask the following questions when considering a treatment facility:

- Has the facility had experience and success in treating my condition?
- Has the facility been rated by state, consumer, or other groups for its quality of care?
- How does the facility check and work to improve its quality of care?
- Has the facility been approved by a nationally recognized accrediting body, such as the American College of Surgeons (ACOS) and/or the Joint Commission on Accredited Healthcare Organizations (JCAHO)?
- Does the facility explain patients' rights and responsibilities? Are copies of this information available to patients?
- Does the treatment facility offer support services, such as social workers and resources to help me find financial assistance if I need it?
- Is the facility conveniently located?

If you are a member of a health insurance plan, your choice of treatment facilities may be limited to those that participate in your plan. Your insurance company can provide you with a list of approved facilities. Although the costs of cancer treatment can be very high, you have the option of paying out-of-pocket if you want to use a treatment facility that is not covered by your insurance plan. If you are considering paying for treatment yourself, you may wish to discuss the potential costs with your doctor beforehand. You may also want to speak with the person who does the billing for the treatment facility. In some instances, nurses and social workers can provide you with more information about coverage, eligibility, and insurance issues.

The following resources may help you find a hospital or treatment facility for your care:

- The NCI fact sheet *The National Cancer Institute Cancer Centers Program* describes and gives contact information for NCI-designated cancer treatment centers around the country.
- The ACOS accredits cancer programs at hospitals and other treatment facilities. More than 1,400 programs in the United States have been designated by the ACOS as Approved Cancer Programs. The ACOS Web site offers a searchable database of these programs at **http://web.facs.org/cpm/default.htm** on the Internet. The ACOS can be

contacted at 633 North Saint Clair Street, Chicago, IL 60611-3211; or by telephone at 312-202-5000.

- The JCAHO is an independent, not-for-profit organization that evaluates and accredits health care organizations and programs in the United States. It also offers information for the general public about choosing a treatment facility. The JCAHO Web site is located at **http://www.jcaho.org** on the Internet. The JCAHO is located at One Renaissance Boulevard, Oakbrook Terrace, IL 60181-4294. The telephone number is 630-792-5800.

- The JCAHO offers an online Quality Check service that patients can use to determine whether a specific facility has been accredited by the JCAHO and view the organization's performance reports. This service is located at **http://www.jcaho.org/qualitycheck/directry/directry.asp** on the Internet.

- The AHRQ publication *Your Guide To Choosing Quality Health Care* has suggestions and checklists for choosing the treatment facility that is right for you.

Additional Cancer Support Information

In addition to the references above, the NCI has set up guidance Web sites that offers information on issues relating to cancer. These include:

- Facing Forward - A Guide for Cancer Survivors:
  http://www.cancer.gov/cancer_information/doc_img.aspx?viewid=cc93a 843-6fc0-409e-8798-5c65afc172fe

- Taking Time: Support for People With Cancer and the People Who Care About Them:
  http://www.cancer.gov/cancer_information/doc_img.aspx?viewid=21a4 6445-a5c8-4fee-95a3-d9d0d665077a

- When Cancer Recurs: Meeting the Challenge:
  http://www.cancer.gov/cancer_information/doc_img.aspx?viewid=9e13 d0d2-b7de-4bd6-87da-5750300a0dab

- Your Health Care Team: Your Doctor Is Only the Beginning:
  http://cis.nci.nih.gov/fact/8_10.htm

Vocabulary Builder

The following vocabulary builder provides definitions of words used in this chapter that have not been defined in previous chapters:

Bereavement: Refers to the whole process of grieving and mourning and is associated with a deep sense of loss and sadness. [NIH]

Bladder: The organ that stores urine. [NIH]

Cervical: Relating to the neck, or to the neck of any organ or structure. Cervical lymph nodes are located in the neck; cervical cancer refers to cancer of the uterine cervix, which is the lower, narrow end (the "neck") of the uterus. [NIH]

Charities: Social welfare organizations with programs designed to assist individuals in times of need. [NIH]

Colon: The long, coiled, tubelike organ that removes water from digested food. The remaining material, solid waste called stool, moves through the colon to the rectum and leaves the body through the anus. [NIH]

Curative: Tending to overcome disease and promote recovery. [EU]

Dermatologist: A doctor who specializes in the diagnosis and treatment of skin problems. [NIH]

Leukemia: Cancer of blood-forming tissue. [NIH]

Lymphoma: Cancer that arises in cells of the lymphatic system. [NIH]

Malignancy: A cancerous tumor that can invade and destroy nearby tissue and spread to other parts of the body. [NIH]

Mammogram: An x-ray of the breast. [NIH]

Mammography: The use of x-rays to create a picture of the breast. [NIH]

Melanosis: A disorder caused by a disturbance in melanin pigmentation; melanism. [EU]

Nevus: A benign growth on the skin, such as a mole. A mole is a cluster of melanocytes and surrounding supportive tissue that usually appears as a tan, brown, or flesh-colored spot on the skin. The plural of nevus is nevi (NEE-vye). [NIH]

Oncologist: A doctor who specializes in treating cancer. Some oncologists specialize in a particular type of cancer treatment. For example, a radiation oncologist specializes in treating cancer with radiation. [NIH]

Palliative: 1. affording relief, but not cure. 2. an alleviating medicine. [EU]

Pancreatic: Having to do with the pancreas. [NIH]

Pap test: The collection of cells from the cervix for examination under a microscope. It is used to detect changes that may be cancer or may lead to cancer, and can show noncancerous conditions, such as infection or inflammation. Also called a Pap smear. [NIH]

Prostate: A gland in males that surrounds the neck of the bladder and the urethra. It secretes a substance that liquifies coagulated semen. It is situated in the pelvic cavity behind the lower part of the pubic symphysis, above the deep layer of the triangular ligament, and rests upon the rectum. [NIH]

Radiologist: A doctor who specializes in creating and interpreting pictures of areas inside the body. The pictures are produced with x-rays, sound waves, or other types of energy. [NIH]

Rectal: By or having to do with the rectum. The rectum is the last 8 to 10 inches of the large intestine and ends at the anus. [NIH]

Screening: Checking for disease when there are no symptoms. [NIH]

Spectrum: A charted band of wavelengths of electromagnetic vibrations obtained by refraction and diffraction. By extension, a measurable range of activity, such as the range of bacteria affected by an antibiotic (antibacterial s.) or the complete range of manifestations of a disease. [EU]

Stomach: An organ that is part of the digestive system. It helps in the digestion of food by mixing it with digestive juices and churning it into a thin liquid. [NIH]

Thyroid: A gland located near the windpipe (trachea) that produces thyroid hormone, which helps regulate growth and metabolism. [NIH]

CHAPTER 3. CLINICAL TRIALS AND MERKEL CELL CARCINOMA

Overview

Very few medical conditions have a single treatment. The basic treatment guidelines that your physician has discussed with you, or those that you have found using the techniques discussed in Chapter 1, may provide you with all that you will require. For some patients, current treatments can be enhanced with new or innovative techniques currently under investigation. In this chapter, we will describe how clinical trials work and show you how to keep informed of trials concerning merkel cell carcinoma.

What Is a Clinical Trial?[17]

Clinical trials involve the participation of people in medical research. Most medical research begins with studies in test tubes and on animals. Treatments that show promise in these early studies may then be tried with people. The only sure way to find out whether a new treatment is safe, effective, and better than other treatments for merkel cell carcinoma is to try it on patients in a clinical trial.

---

[17] The discussion in this chapter has been adapted from the NIH and the NEI: **www.nei.nih.gov/netrials/ctivr.htm**.

What Kinds of Clinical Trials Are There?

Clinical trials are carried out in three phases:

- **Phase I.** Researchers first conduct Phase I trials with small numbers of patients and healthy volunteers. If the new treatment is a medication, researchers also try to determine how much of it can be given safely.
- **Phase II.** Researchers conduct Phase II trials in small numbers of patients to find out the effect of a new treatment on merkel cell carcinoma.
- **Phase III.** Finally, researchers conduct Phase III trials to find out how new treatments for merkel cell carcinoma compare with standard treatments already being used. Phase III trials also help to determine if new treatments have any side effects. These trials--which may involve hundreds, perhaps thousands, of people--can also compare new treatments with no treatment.

How Is a Clinical Trial Conducted?

Various organizations support clinical trials at medical centers, hospitals, universities, and doctors' offices across the United States. The "principal investigator" is the researcher in charge of the study at each facility participating in the clinical trial. Most clinical trial researchers are medical doctors, academic researchers, and specialists. The "clinic coordinator" knows all about how the study works and makes all the arrangements for your visits.

All doctors and researchers who take part in the study on merkel cell carcinoma carefully follow a detailed treatment plan called a protocol. This plan fully explains how the doctors will treat you in the study. The "protocol" ensures that all patients are treated in the same way, no matter where they receive care.

Clinical trials are controlled. This means that researchers compare the effects of the new treatment with those of the standard treatment. In some cases, when no standard treatment exists, the new treatment is compared with no treatment. Patients who receive the new treatment are in the treatment group. Patients who receive a standard treatment or no treatment are in the "control" group. In some clinical trials, patients in the treatment group get a new medication while those in the control group get a placebo. A placebo is a harmless substance, a "dummy" pill, that has no effect on merkel cell carcinoma. In other clinical trials, where a new surgery or device (not a medicine) is being tested, patients in the control group may receive a "sham treatment." This treatment, like a placebo, has no effect on merkel cell carcinoma and does not harm patients.

Researchers assign patients "randomly" to the treatment or control group. This is like flipping a coin to decide which patients are in each group. If you choose to participate in a clinical trial, you will not know which group you will be appointed to. The chance of any patient getting the new treatment is about 50 percent. You cannot request to receive the new treatment instead of the placebo or sham treatment. Often, you will not know until the study is over whether you have been in the treatment group or the control group. This is called a "masked" study. In some trials, neither doctors nor patients know who is getting which treatment. This is called a "double masked" study. These types of trials help to ensure that the perceptions of the patients or doctors will not affect the study results.

Natural History Studies

Unlike clinical trials in which patient volunteers may receive new treatments, natural history studies provide important information to researchers on how merkel cell carcinoma develops over time. A natural history study follows patient volunteers to see how factors such as age, sex, race, or family history might make some people more or less at risk for merkel cell carcinoma. A natural history study may also tell researchers if diet, lifestyle, or occupation affects how a disease or disorder develops and progresses. Results from these studies provide information that helps answer questions such as: How fast will a disease or disorder usually progress? How bad will the condition become? Will treatment be needed?

What Is Expected of Patients in a Clinical Trial?

Not everyone can take part in a clinical trial for a specific disease or disorder. Each study enrolls patients with certain features or eligibility criteria. These criteria may include the type and stage of disease or disorder, as well as, the age and previous treatment history of the patient. You or your doctor can contact the sponsoring organization to find out more about specific clinical trials and their eligibility criteria. If you are interested in joining a clinical trial, your doctor must contact one of the trial's investigators and provide details about your diagnosis and medical history.

If you participate in a clinical trial, you may be required to have a number of medical tests. You may also need to take medications and/or undergo surgery. Depending upon the treatment and the examination procedure, you may be required to receive inpatient hospital care. Or, you may have to return to the medical facility for follow-up examinations. These exams help find out how well the treatment is working. Follow-up studies can take months or years. However, the success of the clinical trial often depends on learning what happens to patients over a long period of time. Only patients who continue to return for follow-up examinations can provide this important long-term information.

Recent Trials on Merkel Cell Carcinoma

The National Institutes of Health and other organizations sponsor trials on various diseases and disorders. Because funding for research goes to the medical areas that show promising research opportunities, it is not possible for the NIH or others to sponsor clinical trials for every disease and disorder at all times. The following lists recent trials dedicated to merkel cell carcinoma.[18] If the trial listed by the NIH is still recruiting, you may be eligible. If it is no longer recruiting or has been completed, then you can contact the sponsors to learn more about the study and, if published, the results. Further information on the trial is available at the Web site indicated. Please note that some trials may no longer be recruiting patients or are otherwise closed. Before contacting sponsors of a clinical trial, consult with your physician who can help you determine if you might benefit from participation.

- **Antineoplaston Therapy in Treating Patients With Neuroendocrine Tumor That Is Metastatic or Unlikely to Respond to Surgery or Radiation Therapy**

    Condition(s): ACTH-producing pituitary tumor; somatostatinoma; nonfunctioning pituitary tumor; TSH producing pituitary tumor; growth hormone-producing pituitary tumor; stage III Merkel cell carcinoma; prolactin-producing pituitary tumor; recurrent Merkel cell carcinoma; neuroendocrine carcinoma; recurrent pituitary tumor

    Study Status: This study is currently recruiting patients.

    Sponsor(s): Burzynski Research Institute

    Purpose - Excerpt: Rationale: Antineoplastons are naturally occurring substances found in urine. Antineoplastons may inhibit the growth of cancer cells. Purpose: Phase II trial to study the effectiveness of antineoplaston therapy in treating patients with neuroendocrine tumor that is metastatic or unlikely to respond to surgery or radiation therapy.

---

[18] These are listed at **www.ClinicalTrials.gov**.

Phase(s): Phase II

Study Type: Treatment

Contact(s): Texas; Burzynski Research Institute, Houston, Texas, 77055, United States; Recruiting; Stanislaw R. Burzynski 713-335-5697. Study chairs or principal investigators: Stanislaw R. Burzynski, Study Chair; Burzynski Research Institute

Web Site:
http://clinicaltrials.gov/ct/gui/show/NCT00003514;jsessionid=9446B0B55BF460F6D2C50B0E804B6395

Benefits and Risks[19]

What Are the Benefits of Participating in a Clinical Trial?

If you are interested in a clinical trial, it is important to realize that your participation can bring many benefits to you and society at large:

- A new treatment could be more effective than the current treatment for merkel cell carcinoma. Although only half of the participants in a clinical trial receive the experimental treatment, if the new treatment is proved to be more effective and safer than the current treatment, then those patients who did not receive the new treatment during the clinical trial may be among the first to benefit from it when the study is over.

- If the treatment is effective, then it may improve health or prevent diseases or disorders.

- Clinical trial patients receive the highest quality of medical care. Experts watch them closely during the study and may continue to follow them after the study is over.

- People who take part in trials contribute to scientific discoveries that may help other people with merkel cell carcinoma. In cases where certain diseases or disorders run in families, your participation may lead to better care or prevention for your family members.

---

[19] This section has been adapted from ClinicalTrials.gov, a service of the National Institutes of Health:
http://www.clinicaltrials.gov/ct/gui/c/a1r/info/whatis?JServSessionIdzone_ct=9jmun6f291.

The Informed Consent

Once you agree to take part in a clinical trial, you will be asked to sign an "informed consent." This document explains a clinical trial's risks and benefits, the researcher's expectations of you, and your rights as a patient.

What Are the Risks?

Clinical trials may involve risks as well as benefits. Whether or not a new treatment will work cannot be known ahead of time. There is always a chance that a new treatment may not work better than a standard treatment. There is also the possibility that it may be harmful. The treatment you receive may cause side effects that are serious enough to require medical attention.

How Is Patient Safety Protected?

Clinical trials can raise fears of the unknown. Understanding the safeguards that protect patients can ease some of these fears. Before a clinical trial begins, researchers must get approval from their hospital's Institutional Review Board (IRB), an advisory group that makes sure a clinical trial is designed to protect patient safety. During a clinical trial, doctors will closely watch you to see if the treatment is working and if you are experiencing any side effects. All the results are carefully recorded and reviewed. In many cases, experts from the Data and Safety Monitoring Committee carefully monitor each clinical trial and can recommend that a study be stopped at any time. You will only be asked to take part in a clinical trial as a volunteer giving informed consent.

What Are a Patient's Rights in a Clinical Trial?

If you are eligible for a clinical trial, you will be given information to help you decide whether or not you want to participate. As a patient, you have the right to:

- Information on all known risks and benefits of the treatments in the study.

- Know how the researchers plan to carry out the study, for how long, and where.

- Know what is expected of you.

- Know any costs involved for you or your insurance provider.
- Know before any of your medical or personal information is shared with other researchers involved in the clinical trial.
- Talk openly with doctors and ask any questions.

After you join a clinical trial, you have the right to:

- Leave the study at any time. Participation is strictly voluntary. However, you should not enroll if you do not plan to complete the study.
- Receive any new information about the new treatment.
- Continue to ask questions and get answers.
- Maintain your privacy. Your name will not appear in any reports based on the study.
- Know whether you participated in the treatment group or the control group (once the study has been completed).

What Should You Ask before Deciding to Join a Clinical Trial?

Questions you should ask when thinking about joining a clinical trial include the following:

- What is the purpose of the clinical trial?
- What are the standard treatments for merkel cell carcinoma? Why do researchers think the new treatment may be better? What is likely to happen to me with or without the new treatment?
- What tests and treatments will I need? Will I need surgery? Medication? Hospitalization?
- How long will the treatment last? How often will I have to come back for follow-up exams?
- What are the treatment's possible benefits to my condition? What are the short- and long-term risks? What are the possible side effects?
- Will the treatment be uncomfortable? Will it make me feel sick? If so, for how long?
- How will my health be monitored?
- Where will I need to go for the clinical trial? How will I get there?
- How much will it cost to be in the study? What costs are covered by the study? How much will my health insurance cover?

- Will I be able to see my own doctor? Who will be in charge of my care?
- Will taking part in the study affect my daily life? Do I have time to participate?
- How do I feel about taking part in a clinical trial? Are there family members or friends who may benefit from my contributions to new medical knowledge?

Clinical Trials and Insurance Coverage[20]

As you consider enrolling in a clinical trial, you will face the critical issue of how to cover the costs of care. Even if you have health insurance, your coverage may not include some or all of the patient care costs associated with a clinical trial. This is because some health plans define clinical trials as "experimental" or "investigational" procedures.

Because lack of coverage for these costs can keep people from enrolling in trials, the National Cancer Institute is working with major health plans and managed care groups to find solutions. In the meantime, there are strategies that may help you deal with cost and coverage barriers. This section answers frequently asked questions about insurance coverage for clinical trial participation and directs you to additional information resources.

The material here is mainly concerned with treatment clinical trials, since other types of trials (prevention, screening, etc.) are newer and generally not covered by health insurance at all. However, this guide may become more relevant for prevention and other types of trials as these trials grow more common.

If you do not have any health insurance, you may find this section helpful for understanding some of the costs that trials involve.

What Costs Do Trials Involve? Who Is Usually Responsible for Paying Them?

There are two types of costs associated with a trial: patient care costs and research costs.
Patient care costs fall into two categories:

---

[20] Adapted from the NCI:
http://www.cancer.gov/clinical_trials/doc_header.aspx?viewid=1d92be79-8748-4bda-8005-2a56d332463b.

- Usual care costs, such as doctor visits, hospital stays, clinical laboratory tests, x-rays, etc., which occur whether you are participating in a trial or receiving standard treatment. These costs have usually been covered by a third-party health plan, such as Medicare or private insurance.
- Extra care costs associated with clinical trial participation, such as the additional tests that may or may not be fully covered by the clinical trial sponsor and/or research institution.

The sponsor and the participant's health plan need to resolve coverage of these costs for particular trials.

Research costs are those associated with conducting the trial, such as data collection and management, research physician and nurse time, analysis of results, and tests purely performed for research purposes. Such costs are usually covered by the sponsoring organization, such as NCI or a pharmaceutical company.

Criteria Used by Health Plans to Make Reimbursement Decisions about Trials

Health insurance companies and managed care companies decide which health care services they will pay for by developing coverage policy regarding the specific services. In general, the most important factor determining whether something is covered is a health plan's judgment as to whether the service is established or investigational. Health plans usually designate a service as established if there is a certain amount of scientific data to show that it is safe and effective. If the health plan does not think that such data exist in sufficient quantity, the plan may label the service as investigational.

Health care services delivered within the setting of a clinical trial are very often categorized as investigational and not covered. This is because the health plan thinks that the major reason to perform the clinical trial is that there is not enough data to establish the safety and effectiveness of the service being studied. Thus, for some health plans, any mention of the fact that the patient is involved in a clinical trial results in a denial of payment.

Your health plan may define specific criteria that a trial must meet before extending coverage, such as the following:

Sponsorship

Some plans may only cover costs of trials sponsored by organizations whose review and oversight of the trial is careful and scientifically rigorous, according to standards set by the health plan.

Trial Phase and Type

Some plans may cover patient care costs only for the clinical trials they judge to be "medically necessary" on a case-by-case basis. Trial phase may also affect coverage; for example, while a plan may be willing to cover costs associated with Phase III trials, which include treatments that have already been successful with a certain number of people, the plan may require some documentation of effectiveness before covering a Phase I or II trial.

While health plans are interested in efforts to improve prevention and screening, they currently seem less likely to have a review process in place for these trials. Therefore, it may be more difficult to get coverage for the care costs associated with them.

Some plans, especially smaller ones, will not cover any costs associated with a clinical trial. Policies vary widely, but in most cases your best bet is to have your doctor initiate discussions with the health plan.

Cost "Neutrality"

Some health plans may limit coverage to trials they consider cost-neutral (i.e., not significantly more expensive than the treatments considered standard).

Lack of Standard Therapy

Some plans limit coverage of trials to situations in which no standard therapy is available.

Facility and Personnel Qualifications

A health plan may require that the facility and medical staff meet specific qualifications to conduct a trial involving unique services, especially intensive therapy such as a bone marrow transplant (high-dose chemotherapy with bone marrow/ stem cell rescue).

Clinical Trials and Medicare Coverage

For up-to-date information about Medicare coverage of clinical trials, go to the Web site for the Centers for Medicaid & Medicare (**http://www.hcfa.gov/coverage/8d.htm**; formerly the Health Care Financing Administration). As of January 2001, the following information was accurate[21]:

What Will Medicare Pay?

- Anything normally covered is still covered when it is part of a clinical trial. This includes test, procedures, and doctor visits that are ordinarily covered.

- Anything normally covered even if it is a service or item associated with the experimental treatment. For example, Medicare will pay for the intravenous administration of a new chemotherapy drug being tested in a trial, including any therapy to prevent side effects from the new drug.

- Anything normally covered even if it resulted from your being in the clinical trial. For example, a test or hospitalization resulting from a side effect of the new treatment that Medicare would ordinarily cover.

What Costs Are Not Covered?

- Investigational items or services being tested in a trial. Sponsors of clinical trials often provide the new drug free, but make sure you ask your doctor before you begin.

- Items or services used solely for the data collection needs of the trial.

- Anything being provided free by the sponsor of the trial.

---

[21] On June 7, 2000, Present Clinton announced that Medicare would revise its payment policy to reimburse the routine patient care costs of clinical trials. The announcement is available for public viewing at the following Web address:
http://www.cancer.gov/clinical_trials/doc.aspx?viewid=320DD013-BA7A-4177-A000-2011089F34A0.

What Kinds of Clinical Trials Are Covered?

NCI's Cancer Information Service has provided a fact sheet for Medicare beneficiaries at the following Web site: **http://cis.nci.nih.gov/fact/8_14.htm**. In general, cancer treatment and diagnosis trials are covered if:

- They are funded by the National Cancer Institute (NCI), NCI-Designated Cancer Centers, NCI-Sponsored Clinical Trials Cooperative Groups and all other Federal agencies that fund cancer research. Other trials may be eligible for coverage and doctors can ask Medicare to pay the patients' costs. Ask your doctor about this before you begin.

- They are designed to treat or diagnose your cancer.

- The purpose or subject of the trial is within a Medicare benefit category. For example, cancer diagnosis and treatment are Medicare benefits, so these trials are covered. Cancer prevention trials are not currently covered.

Increasing the Likelihood of Insurance Coverage for Trials[22]

There are several steps you can follow to deal with coverage issues up front when deciding to enter a clinical trial. Along the way, enlist the help of family members and your doctor or other health professionals. You may find the following checklist useful:

Understand the Costs Associated with the Trial

Ask your doctor or the trial's contact person about the costs that must be covered by you or your health plan. Are these costs significantly higher than those associated with standard care? Also, inquire about the experience of other patients in the trial. Have their plans paid for their care? Have there been any persistent problems with coverage? How often have the trial's administrators been successful in getting plans to cover patient care costs?

---

[22] This section has been adapted from the NCI: http://www.cancer.gov/clinical_trials/doc_header.aspx?viewid=1d92be79-8748-4bda-8005-2a56d332463b&docid=0df4397a-eccb-465f-bd33-a89e7a708c46.

Understand Your Health Plan

Be sure you know what's in your policy; request and carefully review the actual contract language. If there's a specific exclusion for "experimental treatment," look closely at the policy to see how the plan defines such treatment and under what conditions it might be covered. If it is not clearly defined, call the plan's customer service line, consult their Web site, and/or write to them. Ask for specific information about clinical trials coverage.

Work Closely with Your Doctor

Talk with your doctor about the paperwork he or she submits to your health plan. If there have been problems with coverage in the past, you might ask your doctor or the hospital to send an information package to the plan that includes studies supporting the procedure's safety, benefits, and medical appropriateness. This package might include:

- Publications from peer-reviewed literature about the proposed therapy that demonstrate patient benefits;
- A letter that uses the insurance contract's own language to explain why the treatment, screening method, or preventive measure should be covered;
- Letters from researchers that explain the clinical trial;
- Support letters from patient advocacy groups.

Be sure to keep your own copy of any materials that the doctor sends to your health plan for future reference.

Work Closely with Your Company's Benefits Manager

This person may be helpful in enlisting the support of your employer to request coverage by the health plan.

Give Your Health Plan a Deadline

Ask the hospital or cancer center to set a target date for the therapy. This will help to ensure that coverage decisions are made promptly.

Know Your Rights[23]

A number of state governments are addressing the question of whether insurance companies ought to cover the costs associated with patients' participation in clinical trials. Lack of such coverage is a significant barrier to many patients who might otherwise benefit from enrolling in a trial. Lack of coverage also makes it harder for researchers to successfully conduct trials that could improve prevention and treatment options. Information on State initiatives and legislation concerning cancer-related clinical trials is available at **http://www.cancer.gov/ClinicalTrials/insurancelaws**. By conducting your own research and learning about your rights, you may increase the likelihood that your insurance company will cover the costs of a trial.

If Your Insurance Claim Is Denied after the Trial Has Begun

If a claim is denied, read your policy to find out what steps you can follow to make an appeal. In "What Cancer Survivors Need to Know about Health Insurance", the National Coalition for Cancer Survivorship suggests that you and your doctor demonstrate to the health plan that:

- The therapy is not just a research study, but also a valid procedure that benefits patients;
- Your situation is similar to that of other patients who are participating in clinical trials as part of a covered benefit;
- Possible complications have been anticipated and can be handled effectively.

You also may wish to contact your state insurance counseling hotline or insurance department for more help, or write your state insurance commissioner describing the problem.

Where Else Can I Turn for Assistance?

It's never easy to deal with financial issues when you or a loved one faces cancer. Unfortunately, costs can present a significant barrier to clinical trials participation. The range of insurance issues and health plan contracts makes it impossible to deal with all of them here. You may wish to consult this partial list of publications, organizations, and Web sites for more information:

---

[23] Adapted from Cancer.gov: **http://www.cancer.gov/ClinicalTrials/insurancelaws**.

Publications

What Cancer Survivors Need to Know about Health Insurance
National Coalition of Cancer Survivorship
1010 Wayne Avenue, 5th floor
Silver Spring, MD 20910
(301) 650-8868
http://www.cansearch.org/

Cancer Treatments Your Insurance Should Cover
The Association of Community Cancer Centers
11600 Nebel Street, Suite 201
Rockville, MD 20852
(301) 984-9496
http://www.accc-cancer.org/main2001.shtml

The Managed Care Answer Guide
Patient Advocate Foundation
739 Thimble Shoals Boulevard, Suite 704
Newport News, VA 23606
(757) 873-6668
E-mail: **ndepaf@pinn.net**

1998 Guide to Health Insurance for People with Medicare, The Medicare Handbook
Medicare Helpline: 1-800-444-4606
Health Care Financing Administration: **http://www.hcfa.gov/**
New Medicare site: **http://www.medicare.gov/**

Assistance Programs

Candlelighters Childhood Cancer Foundation
Ombudsman Program
910 Woodmont Avenue, #4607
Bethesda, MD 20814
(301) 657-8401; 1-800-366-2223 (toll-free)
E-mail: **info@candlelighters.org**
http://www.candlelighters.org
The Ombudsman Program helps families of children with cancer and survivors of childhood cancer resolve a range of problems, including insurance coverage difficulties. Local groups appoint a Parent Advocate who works with the treatment center on behalf of families.

Medical Care Management Corporation
5272 River Road, Suite 650
Bethesda, MD 20816-1405
(301) 652-1818
email: mcman@mcman.com
http://www.mcman.com/
Working for a range of clients, including health plans, employers, and patients, MCMC conducts independent, objective reviews of high-technology medical care cases to assist in decision-making. While it does charge for its services, MCMC also offers a volunteer program for those who cannot afford to pay.

More Information Resources

OncoLink
A service of the University of Pennsylvania Cancer Center.
http://www.oncolink.com/
In addition to general cancer information, this web site features a section on financial information for patients. Among the topics: viatical settlements, life insurance, a glossary of financial and medical terms, and news about billing and insurance.

American Association of Health Plans
1129 20th Street, NW, Suite 600
Washington, DC 20036-3421
(202) 778-3200
http://www.aahp.org/
The Web site section "For Consumers" includes a fact sheet on clinical research that describes various health plans' efforts to support research initiatives and collaborate with academic health centers and universities.

Health Insurance Association of America
555 13th Street, NW
Washington, DC 20004
(202) 824-1600

- Home page: http://www.hiaa.org/

- Consumer Information: http://www.hiaa.org/consumer/

- Insurance Counseling Hotlines by State:
  http://www.hiaa.org/consumer/insurance_counsel.cfm

- State Insurance Departments:
  http://www.hiaa.org/consumer/state_insurance.cfm

Government Initiatives to Expand Insurance Coverage for Trials[24]

The good news is that there has been a recent effort in the U.S. to assure clinical trials coverage, with NCI involved in several new initiatives as described below:

NCI-Department of Defense Agreement

An innovative 1996 agreement between NCI and the Department of Defense (DoD) has given thousands of DoD cancer patients more options for care and greater access to state-of-the-art treatments. Patients who are beneficiaries of TRICARE/CHAMPUS, the DoD's health program, are covered for NCI-sponsored Phase II and Phase III clinical treatment trials. NCI and DoD are refining a system that allows physicians and patients to determine quickly what current trials meet their needs and where they are taking place.

NCI-Department of Veterans Affairs Agreement

A 1997 agreement with the Department of Veterans Affairs provides coverage for eligible veterans of the armed services to participate in NCI-sponsored prevention, diagnosis, and treatment studies nationwide. For additional information, see the VA/DoD Beneficiaries Digest Page at http://www.va.gov/cancer.htm.

Midwest Health Plans Agreement

Some NCI Cooperative Groups have reached agreements with several insurers in Wisconsin and Minnesota to provide more than 200,000 people with coverage. This coverage is allocated for patient care costs if they participate in a cooperative group-sponsored trial.

---

[24] Adapted from the NCI:
http://www.cancer.gov/clinical_trials/doc_header.aspx?viewid=1d92be79-8748-4bda-8005-2a56d332463b&docid=d8092601-daf9-4794-8536-3be2712eb6b9.

Pediatric Cancer Care Network

This network, a cooperative agreement among the Children's Cancer Group, the Pediatric Oncology Group, and the Blue Cross Blue Shield System Association (BCBS) nationwide, will ensure that children of BCBS subscribers receive care at designated centers of cancer care excellence and may promote the enrollment of children in Cooperative Group clinical trials.

Keeping Current on Clinical Trials

Various government agencies maintain databases on trials. The U.S. National Institutes of Health, through the National Library of Medicine, has developed ClinicalTrials.gov to provide patients, family members, and physicians with current information about clinical research across the broadest number of diseases and conditions.

The site was launched in February 2000 and currently contains approximately 5,700 clinical studies in over 59,000 locations worldwide, with most studies being conducted in the United States. ClinicalTrials.gov receives about 2 million hits per month and hosts approximately 5,400 visitors daily. To access this database, simply go to their Web site (**www.clinicaltrials.gov**) and search by "merkel cell carcinoma" (or synonyms).

While ClinicalTrials.gov is the most comprehensive listing of NIH-supported clinical trials available, not all trials are in the database. The database is updated regularly, so clinical trials are continually being added. The following is a list of specialty databases affiliated with the National Institutes of Health that offer additional information on trials:

- For clinical studies at the Warren Grant Magnuson Clinical Center located in Bethesda, Maryland, visit their Web site:
  http://clinicalstudies.info.nih.gov/

- For clinical studies conducted at the Bayview Campus in Baltimore, Maryland, visit their Web site:
  http://www.jhbmc.jhu.edu/studies/index.html

- For cancer trials, visit the National Cancer Institute:
  http://cancertrials.nci.nih.gov/

General References

The following references describe clinical trials and experimental medical research. They have been selected to ensure that they are likely to be available from your local or online bookseller or university medical library. These references are usually written for healthcare professionals, so you may consider consulting with a librarian or bookseller who might recommend a particular reference. The following includes some of the most readily available references (sorted alphabetically by title; hyperlinks provide rankings, information and reviews at Amazon.com):

- **A Guide to Patient Recruitment : Today's Best Practices & Proven Strategies** by Diana L. Anderson; Paperback - 350 pages (2001), CenterWatch, Inc.; ISBN: 1930624115;
  http://www.amazon.com/exec/obidos/ASIN/1930624115/icongroupinterna

- **A Step-By-Step Guide to Clinical Trials** by Marilyn Mulay, R.N., M.S., OCN; Spiral-bound - 143 pages Spiral edition (2001), Jones & Bartlett Pub; ISBN: 0763715697;
  http://www.amazon.com/exec/obidos/ASIN/0763715697/icongroupinterna

- **The CenterWatch Directory of Drugs in Clinical Trials** by CenterWatch; Paperback - 656 pages (2000), CenterWatch, Inc.; ISBN: 0967302935;
  http://www.amazon.com/exec/obidos/ASIN/0967302935/icongroupinterna

- **The Complete Guide to Informed Consent in Clinical Trials** by Terry Hartnett (Editor); Paperback - 164 pages (2000), PharmSource Information Services, Inc.; ISBN: 0970153309;
  http://www.amazon.com/exec/obidos/ASIN/0970153309/icongroupinterna

- **Dictionary for Clinical Trials** by Simon Day; Paperback - 228 pages (1999), John Wiley & Sons; ISBN: 0471985961;
  http://www.amazon.com/exec/obidos/ASIN/0471985961/icongroupinterna

- **Extending Medicare Reimbursement in Clinical Trials** by Institute of Medicine Staff (Editor), et al; Paperback 1st edition (2000), National Academy Press; ISBN: 0309068886;
  http://www.amazon.com/exec/obidos/ASIN/0309068886/icongroupinterna

- **Handbook of Clinical Trials** by Marcus Flather (Editor); Paperback (2001), Remedica Pub Ltd; ISBN: 1901346293;
  http://www.amazon.com/exec/obidos/ASIN/1901346293/icongroupinterna

Vocabulary Builder

The following vocabulary builder gives definitions of words used in this chapter that have not been defined in previous chapters:

ACTH: Adrenocorticotropic hormone. [EU]

Antineoplastons: Substances isolated from normal human blood and urine being tested as a type of treatment for some tumors and AIDS. [NIH]

Intravenous: IV. Into a vein. [NIH]

Metastatic: Having to do with metastasis, which is the spread of cancer from one part of the body to another. [NIH]

Prolactin: Pituitary lactogenic hormone. A polypeptide hormone with a molecular weight of about 23,000. It is essential in the induction of lactation in mammals at parturition and is synergistic with estrogen. The hormone also brings about the release of progesterone from lutein cells, which renders the uterine mucosa suited for the embedding of the ovum should fertilization occur. [NIH]

Urine: Fluid containing water and waste products. Urine is made by the kidneys, stored in the bladder, and leaves the body through the urethra. [NIH]

PART II: ADDITIONAL RESOURCES AND ADVANCED MATERIAL

ABOUT PART II

In Part II, we introduce you to additional resources and advanced research on merkel cell carcinoma. All too often, patients who conduct their own research are overwhelmed by the difficulty in finding and organizing information. The purpose of the following chapters is to provide you an organized and structured format to help you find additional information resources on merkel cell carcinoma. In Part II, as in Part I, our objective is not to interpret the latest advances on merkel cell carcinoma or render an opinion. Rather, our goal is to give you access to original research and to increase your awareness of sources you may not have already considered. In this way, you will come across the advanced materials often referred to in pamphlets, books, or other general works. Once again, some of this material is technical in nature, so consultation with a professional familiar with merkel cell carcinoma is suggested.

CHAPTER 4. STUDIES ON MERKEL CELL CARCINOMA

Overview

Every year, academic studies are published on merkel cell carcinoma or related conditions. Broadly speaking, there are two types of studies. The first are peer reviewed. Generally, the content of these studies has been reviewed by scientists or physicians. Peer-reviewed studies are typically published in scientific journals and are usually available at medical libraries. The second type of studies is non-peer reviewed. These works include summary articles that do not use or report scientific results. These often appear in the popular press, newsletters, or similar periodicals.

In this chapter, we will show you how to locate peer-reviewed references and studies on merkel cell carcinoma. We will begin by discussing research that has been summarized and is free to view by the public via the Internet. We then show you how to generate a bibliography on merkel cell carcinoma and teach you how to keep current on new studies as they are published or undertaken by the scientific community.

Federally Funded Research on Merkel Cell Carcinoma

The U.S. Government supports a variety of research studies relating to merkel cell carcinoma and associated conditions. These studies are tracked by the Office of Extramural Research at the National Institutes of Health.[25]

---

[25] Healthcare projects are funded by the National Institutes of Health (NIH), Substance Abuse and Mental Health Services (SAMHSA), Health Resources and Services Administration (HRSA), Food and Drug Administration (FDA), Centers for Disease Control

CRISP (Computerized Retrieval of Information on Scientific Projects) is a searchable database of federally funded biomedical research projects conducted at universities, hospitals, and other institutions. Visit the CRISP Web site at **http://commons.cit.nih.gov/crisp3/CRISP.Generate_Ticket**. You can perform targeted searches by various criteria including geography, date, as well as topics related to merkel cell carcinoma and related conditions.

For most of the studies, the agencies reporting into CRISP provide summaries or abstracts. As opposed to clinical trial research using patients, many federally funded studies use animals or simulated models to explore merkel cell carcinoma and related conditions. In some cases, therefore, it may be difficult to understand how some basic or fundamental research could eventually translate into medical practice. The following sample is typical of the type of information found when searching the CRISP database for merkel cell carcinoma:

- **Project Title: Development of Mechanoreceptors--Role of Neurotrophins**

    Principal Investigator & Institution: Szeder, Viktor; Cell Biol, Neurobiol/Anatomy; Medical College of Wisconsin 8701 Watertown Plank Rd Milwaukee, Wi 53226

    Timing: Fiscal Year 2000; Project Start 5-AUG-2000

    Summary: Merkel cells are slowly adapting sensory receptors in the skin that are innervated by Abeta sensory neurons. Virtually nothing is known about the cellular and molecular mechanisms that control development and innervation of Merkel cells. My advisor, Prof. Grim, and his collaborators have shown that Merkel cells are derived from the neural crest and that their precursors migrate in the ventrolateral migratory pathway in the subectodermal space. The proposed work is designed to elucidate some of the roles growth factors play in the development of quail neural crest cells into Merkel cells. In Aim 1, Merkel cells in culture will be characterized at the ultrastructural level and compared to Merkel cells in the intact organism. In Aim 2, the expression during embryonic development of pertinent growth factor receptors by Merkel cell precursors and maturing Merkel cells will be elucidated by indirect immunohistochemistry and in situ hybridization. Additionally, the autocrine and/or paracrine expression of the receptor ligands will be determined. Candidate growth factors include stem cell factor (SCF), epidermal growth factor (EGF), nerve growth factor (NGF) and neurotrophin-3 (NT-3). By use of the neural crest cell colony assay

---

and Prevention (CDCP), Agency for Healthcare Research and Quality (AHRQ), and Office of Assistant Secretary of Health (OASH).

that has been developed in Prof. Sieber-Blum's laboratory, I propose in Aim 3 to assess the role of pertinent growth factors (as determined in Aim 2) in the survival, proliferation and differentiation of Merkel cells. The proposed work has relevance to human neurological disease. In individuals with anhidrotic ectodermal dysplasia, and in the corresponding mouse model, Tabby, there are no Merkel cells (Srivastava et al., 1997; Vielkind et al., 1995). This is most likely due to down-regulation of the EGF receptor. In vitiligo, Merkel cells as well as melanocytes are lost (Kumar Bose, 1994). A disrupted neurotrophin-3 gene in mice causes perinatal loss of Merkel cells and other neurodegenerative symptoms (Airaksinen et al., 1996). Merkel cell carcinoma (small, intermediate and trabecular types) is a relatively frequent tumor (Schmidt et al., 1998). Insights into the mechanisms that regulate normal Merkel cell development may prove useful in future approaches for the prevention or treatment of neurological disease.

Website: http://commons.cit.nih.gov/crisp3/CRISP.Generate_Ticket

E-Journals: PubMed Central[26]

PubMed Central (PMC) is a digital archive of life sciences journal literature developed and managed by the National Center for Biotechnology Information (NCBI) at the U.S. National Library of Medicine (NLM).[27] Access to this growing archive of e-journals is free and unrestricted.[28] To search, go to **http://www.pubmedcentral.nih.gov/index.html#search**, and type "merkel cell carcinoma" (or synonyms) into the search box. This search gives you access to full-text articles. The following is a sample of items found for merkel cell carcinoma in the PubMed Central database:

- **Comparison of Mutant and Wild-Type p53 Proteins in Merkel Cell Carcinoma** by Henry J. Carson, Nathan E. Lueck, and Bruce C. Horten; 2000 March
  http://www.pubmedcentral.nih.gov/articlerender.fcgi?artid=95873

---

[26] Adapted from the National Library of Medicine: **http://www.pubmedcentral.nih.gov/about/intro.html**.

[27] With PubMed Central, NCBI is taking the lead in preservation and maintenance of open access to electronic literature, just as NLM has done for decades with printed biomedical literature. PubMed Central aims to become a world-class library of the digital age.

[28] The value of PubMed Central, in addition to its role as an archive, lies the availability of data from diverse sources stored in a common format in a single repository. Many journals already have online publishing operations, and there is a growing tendency to publish material online only, to the exclusion of print.

The National Library of Medicine: PubMed

One of the quickest and most comprehensive ways to find academic studies in both English and other languages is to use PubMed, maintained by the National Library of Medicine. The advantage of PubMed over previously mentioned sources is that it covers a greater number of domestic and foreign references. It is also free to the public.[29] If the publisher has a Web site that offers full text of its journals, PubMed will provide links to that site, as well as to sites offering other related data. User registration, a subscription fee, or some other type of fee may be required to access the full text of articles in some journals.

To generate your own bibliography of studies dealing with merkel cell carcinoma, simply go to the PubMed Web site at **www.ncbi.nlm.nih.gov/pubmed**. Type "merkel cell carcinoma" (or synonyms) into the search box, and click "Go." The following is the type of output you can expect from PubMed for "merkel cell carcinoma" (hyperlinks lead to article summaries):

- **123I-MIBG SPECT of Merkel cell carcinoma.**
  Author(s): Watanabe N, Shimizu M, Kageyama M, Kitagawa K, Hayasaka S, Seto H.
  Source: The British Journal of Radiology. 1998 August; 71(848): 886-7.
  http://www.ncbi.nlm.nih.gov:80/entrez/query.fcgi?cmd=Retrieve&db=PubMed&list_uids=9828805&dopt=Abstract

- **A case of Merkel cell carcinoma with extension into the orbital cavity.**
  Author(s): Yildirim S, Akoz T, Yavuzer D, Akan M, Avci G.
  Source: Annals of Plastic Surgery. 2001 February; 46(2): 198-9. No Abstract Available.
  http://www.ncbi.nlm.nih.gov:80/entrez/query.fcgi?cmd=Retrieve&db=PubMed&list_uids=11216630&dopt=Abstract

- **A case of Merkel cell carcinoma with parotid lymph node metastasis.**
  Author(s): Batman C, Sav A, Mamikoglu B, Uneri C.

---

[29] PubMed was developed by the National Center for Biotechnology Information (NCBI) at the National Library of Medicine (NLM) at the National Institutes of Health (NIH). The PubMed database was developed in conjunction with publishers of biomedical literature as a search tool for accessing literature citations and linking to full-text journal articles at Web sites of participating publishers. Publishers that participate in PubMed supply NLM with their citations electronically prior to or at the time of publication.

Source: Ear, Nose, & Throat Journal. 1994 June; 73(6): 418-9.
http://www.ncbi.nlm.nih.gov:80/entrez/query.fcgi?cmd=Retrieve&db=PubMed&list_uids=8076544&dopt=Abstract

- **A case of rapidly recurring cheek Merkel cell carcinoma.**
  Author(s): Yamamoto T, Akita S, Koga S, Fujii T.
  Source: Annals of Plastic Surgery. 2000 March; 44(3): 349-50. No Abstract Available.
  http://www.ncbi.nlm.nih.gov:80/entrez/query.fcgi?cmd=Retrieve&db=PubMed&list_uids=10735237&dopt=Abstract

- **A Merkel cell carcinoma of the skin.**
  Author(s): Reiffers-Mettelock J, Ries F.
  Source: Bull Soc Sci Med Grand Duche Luxemb. 2001; (1): 39-45.
  http://www.ncbi.nlm.nih.gov:80/entrez/query.fcgi?cmd=Retrieve&db=PubMed&list_uids=11570212&dopt=Abstract

- **A Meta-analysis of the Prognostic Significance of Sentinel Lymph Node Status in Merkel Cell Carcinoma.**
  Author(s): Mehrany K, Otley CC, Weenig RH, Phillips PK, Roenigk RK, Nguyen TH.
  Source: Dermatologic Surgery : Official Publication for American Society for Dermatologic Surgery [et Al.]. 2002 February; 28(2): 113-7.
  http://www.ncbi.nlm.nih.gov:80/entrez/query.fcgi?cmd=Retrieve&db=PubMed&list_uids=11860419&dopt=Abstract

- **A nonconsensus octamer-recognition sequence (TAATGARAT-motif) identifies a novel DNA binding protein in human Merkel cell carcinoma cell lines.**
  Author(s): Thomson JA, Leonard JH, McGregor K, Sturm RA, Parsons PG.
  Source: International Journal of Cancer. Journal International Du Cancer. 1994 July 15; 58(2): 285-90.
  http://www.ncbi.nlm.nih.gov:80/entrez/query.fcgi?cmd=Retrieve&db=PubMed&list_uids=8026890&dopt=Abstract

- **A review of Merkel cell carcinoma with emphasis on lymph node disease in the absence of a primary site.**
  Author(s): Straka JA, Straka MB.

Source: American Journal of Otolaryngology. 1997 January-February; 18(1): 55-65. Review. No Abstract Available.
http://www.ncbi.nlm.nih.gov:80/entrez/query.fcgi?cmd=Retrieve&db=PubMed&list_uids=9006679&dopt=Abstract

- **A study of apoptosis in Merkel cell carcinoma: an immunohistochemical, ultrastructural, DNA ladder, and TUNEL labeling study.**
  Author(s): Mori Y, Hashimoto K, Tanaka K, Cui CY, Mehregan DR, Stiff MA.
  Source: The American Journal of Dermatopathology. 2001 February; 23(1): 16-23.
  http://www.ncbi.nlm.nih.gov:80/entrez/query.fcgi?cmd=Retrieve&db=PubMed&list_uids=11176047&dopt=Abstract

- **Aberrant FHIT transcripts in Merkel cell carcinoma.**
  Author(s): Sozzi G, Alder H, Tornielli S, Corletto V, Baffa R, Veronese ML, Negrini M, Pilotti S, Pierotti MA, Huebner K, Croce CM.
  Source: Cancer Research. 1996 June 1; 56(11): 2472-4.
  http://www.ncbi.nlm.nih.gov:80/entrez/query.fcgi?cmd=Retrieve&db=PubMed&list_uids=8653678&dopt=Abstract

- **Aggressive surgical management for Merkel cell carcinoma.**
  Author(s): Gray LN.
  Source: Plastic and Reconstructive Surgery. 1995 July; 96(1): 237. No Abstract Available.
  http://www.ncbi.nlm.nih.gov:80/entrez/query.fcgi?cmd=Retrieve&db=PubMed&list_uids=7604120&dopt=Abstract

- **Alterations of the SDHD gene locus in midgut carcinoids, Merkel cell carcinomas, pheochromocytomas, and abdominal paragangliomas.**
  Author(s): Kytola S, Nord B, Elder EE, Carling T, Kjellman M, Cedermark B, Juhlin C, Hoog A, Isola J, Larsson C.
  Source: Genes, Chromosomes & Cancer. 2002 July; 34(3): 325-32.
  http://www.ncbi.nlm.nih.gov:80/entrez/query.fcgi?cmd=Retrieve&db=PubMed&list_uids=12007193&dopt=Abstract

- **Ampullary somatostatinoma in a patient with Merkel cell carcinoma.**
  Author(s): Fincher RK, Christensen ED, Tsuchida AM.

Source: The American Journal of Gastroenterology. 1999 July; 94(7): 1955-7.
http://www.ncbi.nlm.nih.gov:80/entrez/query.fcgi?cmd=Retrieve&db=PubMed&list_uids=10406267&dopt=Abstract

- **An unusual pattern of metastases from Merkel cell carcinoma.**
  Author(s): Foster R, Stevens G, Egan M.
  Source: Australasian Radiology. 1994 August; 38(3): 231-2.
  http://www.ncbi.nlm.nih.gov:80/entrez/query.fcgi?cmd=Retrieve&db=PubMed&list_uids=7945123&dopt=Abstract

- **Analysis of thyroid transcription factor-1 and cytokeratin 20 separates merkel cell carcinoma from small cell carcinoma of lung.**
  Author(s): Hanly AJ, Elgart GW, Jorda M, Smith J, Nadji M.
  Source: Journal of Cutaneous Pathology. 2000 March; 27(3): 118-20.
  http://www.ncbi.nlm.nih.gov:80/entrez/query.fcgi?cmd=Retrieve&db=PubMed&list_uids=10728812&dopt=Abstract

- **Anti-Hu antibodies in Merkel cell carcinoma.**
  Author(s): Greenlee JE, Steffens JD, Clawson SA, Hill K, Dalmau J.
  Source: Annals of Neurology. 2002 July; 52(1): 111-5.
  http://www.ncbi.nlm.nih.gov:80/entrez/query.fcgi?cmd=Retrieve&db=PubMed&list_uids=12112058&dopt=Abstract

- **Bcl-2 antisense oligonucleotides (G3139) inhibit Merkel cell carcinoma growth in SCID mice.**
  Author(s): Schlagbauer-Wadl H, Klosner G, Heere-Ress E, Waltering S, Moll I, Wolff K, Pehamberger H, Jansen B.
  Source: The Journal of Investigative Dermatology. 2000 April; 114(4): 725-30.
  http://www.ncbi.nlm.nih.gov:80/entrez/query.fcgi?cmd=Retrieve&db=PubMed&list_uids=10733680&dopt=Abstract

- **Brain metastasis of Merkel cell carcinoma.**
  Author(s): Turgut M.
  Source: Neurosurgical Review. 2002 March; 25(1-2): 113-4. No Abstract Available.
  http://www.ncbi.nlm.nih.gov:80/entrez/query.fcgi?cmd=Retrieve&db=PubMed&list_uids=11954765&dopt=Abstract

- **Brain metastasis of Merkel cell carcinoma. Case report and review of the literature.**

Author(s): Ikawa F, Kiya K, Uozumi T, Yuki K, Takeshita S, Hamasaki O, Arita K, Kurisu K.
Source: Neurosurgical Review. 1999; 22(1): 54-7. Review.
http://www.ncbi.nlm.nih.gov:80/entrez/query.fcgi?cmd=Retrieve&db=PubMed&list_uids=10348209&dopt=Abstract

- **Breast metastases of Merkel cell carcinoma.**
  Author(s): Schnabel T, Glag M.
  Source: European Journal of Cancer (Oxford, England : 1990). 1996 August; 32A(9): 1617-8. No Abstract Available.
  http://www.ncbi.nlm.nih.gov:80/entrez/query.fcgi?cmd=Retrieve&db=PubMed&list_uids=8911130&dopt=Abstract

- **CD117 (KIT Receptor) Expression in Merkel Cell Carcinoma.**
  Author(s): Su LD, Fullen DR, Lowe L, Uherova P, Schnitzer B, Valdez R.
  Source: The American Journal of Dermatopathology. 2002 August; 24(4): 289-93.
  http://www.ncbi.nlm.nih.gov:80/entrez/query.fcgi?cmd=Retrieve&db=PubMed&list_uids=12142606&dopt=Abstract

- **CD44 expression in Merkel cell carcinoma may correlate with risk of metastasis.**
  Author(s): Penneys NS, Shapiro S.
  Source: Journal of Cutaneous Pathology. 1994 February; 21(1): 22-6.
  http://www.ncbi.nlm.nih.gov:80/entrez/query.fcgi?cmd=Retrieve&db=PubMed&list_uids=7514617&dopt=Abstract

- **Characterisation of four Merkel cell carcinoma adherent cell lines.**
  Author(s): Leonard JH, Dash P, Holland P, Kearsley JH, Bell JR.
  Source: International Journal of Cancer. Journal International Du Cancer. 1995 January 3; 60(1): 100-7.
  http://www.ncbi.nlm.nih.gov:80/entrez/query.fcgi?cmd=Retrieve&db=PubMed&list_uids=7814141&dopt=Abstract

- **Characteristic pattern of chromosomal gains and losses in Merkel cell carcinoma detected by comparative genomic hybridization.**
  Author(s): Van Gele M, Speleman F, Vandesompele J, Van Roy N, Leonard JH.
  Source: Cancer Research. 1998 April 1; 58(7): 1503-8.
  http://www.ncbi.nlm.nih.gov:80/entrez/query.fcgi?cmd=Retrieve&db=PubMed&list_uids=9537255&dopt=Abstract

- **Chemotherapy for patients with locally advanced or metastatic Merkel cell carcinoma.**
  Author(s): Voog E, Biron P, Martin JP, Blay JY.
  Source: Cancer. 1999 June 15; 85(12): 2589-95.
  http://www.ncbi.nlm.nih.gov:80/entrez/query.fcgi?cmd=Retrieve&db=PubMed&list_uids=10375107&dopt=Abstract

- **Chemotherapy in neuroendocrine/Merkel cell carcinoma of the skin: case series and review of 204 cases.**
  Author(s): Tai PT, Yu E, Winquist E, Hammond A, Stitt L, Tonita J, Gilchrist J.
  Source: Journal of Clinical Oncology : Official Journal of the American Society of Clinical Oncology. 2000 June; 18(12): 2493-9. Review.
  http://www.ncbi.nlm.nih.gov:80/entrez/query.fcgi?cmd=Retrieve&db=PubMed&list_uids=10856110&dopt=Abstract

- **Chromosomal evolution in a Merkel cell carcinoma.**
  Author(s): Schlegelberger B, Bartels H, Sterry W.
  Source: Cancer Genetics and Cytogenetics. 1994 July 1; 75(1): 74-6. No Abstract Available.
  http://www.ncbi.nlm.nih.gov:80/entrez/query.fcgi?cmd=Retrieve&db=PubMed&list_uids=8039170&dopt=Abstract

- **Chromosome 6 trisomy as sole anomaly in a primary Merkel cell carcinoma.**
  Author(s): Larsimont D, Verhest A.
  Source: Virchows Archiv : an International Journal of Pathology. 1996 July; 428(4-5): 305-9.
  http://www.ncbi.nlm.nih.gov:80/entrez/query.fcgi?cmd=Retrieve&db=PubMed&list_uids=8764942&dopt=Abstract

- **Chromosomes 1, 11, and 13 are frequently involved in karyotypic abnormalities in metastatic Merkel cell carcinoma.**
  Author(s): Leonard JH, Leonard P, Kearsley JH.
  Source: Cancer Genetics and Cytogenetics. 1993 May; 67(1): 65-70.
  http://www.ncbi.nlm.nih.gov:80/entrez/query.fcgi?cmd=Retrieve&db=PubMed&list_uids=8504402&dopt=Abstract

- **Clinical approach to neuroendocrine carcinoma of the skin (Merkel cell carcinoma).**
  Author(s): Smith DF, Messina JL, Perrott R, Berman CG, Reintgen DS, Cruse CW, Glass FL, Fenske NA, DeConti RC, Trotti A 3rd.

Source: Cancer Control : Journal of the Moffitt Cancer Center. 2000 January-February; 7(1): 72-83. Review. No Abstract Available.
http://www.ncbi.nlm.nih.gov:80/entrez/query.fcgi?cmd=Retrieve&db=PubMed&list_uids=10740663&dopt=Abstract

- **Clinical management and treatment outcomes of Merkel cell carcinoma.**
  Author(s): Wong KC, Zuletta F, Clarke SJ, Kennedy PJ.
  Source: The Australian and New Zealand Journal of Surgery. 1998 May; 68(5): 354-8.
  http://www.ncbi.nlm.nih.gov:80/entrez/query.fcgi?cmd=Retrieve&db=PubMed&list_uids=9631909&dopt=Abstract

- **Combined karyotyping, CGH and M-FISH analysis allows detailed characterization of unidentified chromosomal rearrangements in Merkel cell carcinoma.**
  Author(s): Van Gele M, Leonard JH, Van Roy N, Van Limbergen H, Van Belle S, Cocquyt V, Salwen H, De Paepe A, Speleman F.
  Source: International Journal of Cancer. Journal International Du Cancer. 2002 September 10; 101(2): 137-45. Review.
  http://www.ncbi.nlm.nih.gov:80/entrez/query.fcgi?cmd=Retrieve&db=PubMed&list_uids=12209990&dopt=Abstract

- **Comments on the use of sentinel lymph node biopsy in patients with Merkel cell carcinoma.**
  Author(s): Klein AW.
  Source: Dermatologic Surgery : Official Publication for American Society for Dermatologic Surgery [et Al.]. 2000 June; 26(6): 609. No Abstract Available.
  http://www.ncbi.nlm.nih.gov:80/entrez/query.fcgi?cmd=Retrieve&db=PubMed&list_uids=10848952&dopt=Abstract

- **Comparative genomic hybridization (CGH) discloses chromosomal and subchromosomal copy number changes in Merkel cell carcinomas.**
  Author(s): Harle M, Arens N, Moll I, Back W, Schulz T, Scherthan H.
  Source: Journal of Cutaneous Pathology. 1996 October; 23(5): 391-7.
  http://www.ncbi.nlm.nih.gov:80/entrez/query.fcgi?cmd=Retrieve&db=PubMed&list_uids=8915847&dopt=Abstract

- **Comparison of mutant and wild-type p53 proteins in Merkel cell carcinoma.**
  Author(s): Carson HJ, Lueck NE, Horten BC.

Source: Clinical and Diagnostic Laboratory Immunology. 2000 March; 7(2): 326. No Abstract Available.
http://www.ncbi.nlm.nih.gov:80/entrez/query.fcgi?cmd=Retrieve&db=PubMed&list_uids=10798862&dopt=Abstract

- **Complete spontaneous regression of Merkel cell carcinoma: a review of the 10 reported cases.**
  Author(s): Connelly TJ, Cribier B, Brown TJ, Yanguas I.
  Source: Dermatologic Surgery : Official Publication for American Society for Dermatologic Surgery [et Al.]. 2000 September; 26(9): 853-6. Review.
  http://www.ncbi.nlm.nih.gov:80/entrez/query.fcgi?cmd=Retrieve&db=PubMed&list_uids=10971559&dopt=Abstract

- **Computed tomography evaluation of recurrent Merkel cell carcinoma.**
  Author(s): Orr LA, Sotile SC, Byram BR, Brogdon BG.
  Source: Clinical Imaging. 1992 January-March; 16(1): 52-4.
  http://www.ncbi.nlm.nih.gov:80/entrez/query.fcgi?cmd=Retrieve&db=PubMed&list_uids=1540865&dopt=Abstract

- **Cutaneous lymphoma-simulating Merkel cell carcinoma-molecular genetic demonstration of a clonal disease with divergent immunophenotypes.**
  Author(s): Miettinen M, Lasota J.
  Source: Modern Pathology : an Official Journal of the United States and Canadian Academy of Pathology, Inc. 1995 September; 8(7): 769-74.
  http://www.ncbi.nlm.nih.gov:80/entrez/query.fcgi?cmd=Retrieve&db=PubMed&list_uids=8539236&dopt=Abstract

- **Cystic metastasis of the pancreas indicating relapse of Merkel cell carcinoma.**
  Author(s): Bachmeyer C, Alovor G, Chatelain D, Khuoy L, Turc Y, Danon O, Laurette F, Cazier A, N'Guyen V.
  Source: Pancreas. 2002 January; 24(1): 103-5. No Abstract Available.
  http://www.ncbi.nlm.nih.gov:80/entrez/query.fcgi?cmd=Retrieve&db=PubMed&list_uids=11741190&dopt=Abstract

- **Cytokeratin 20: a marker for diagnosing Merkel cell carcinoma.**
  Author(s): Scott MP, Helm KF.

Source: The American Journal of Dermatopathology. 1999 February; 21(1): 16-20.

http://www.ncbi.nlm.nih.gov:80/entrez/query.fcgi?cmd=Retrieve&db=PubMed&list_uids=10027519&dopt=Abstract

- **Cytokeratin and neurofilament protein staining in Merkel cell carcinoma of the small cell type and small cell carcinoma of the lung.**
  Author(s): Schmidt U, Muller U, Metz KA, Leder LD.
  Source: The American Journal of Dermatopathology. 1998 August; 20(4): 346-51.
  http://www.ncbi.nlm.nih.gov:80/entrez/query.fcgi?cmd=Retrieve&db=PubMed&list_uids=9700371&dopt=Abstract

- **Cytokeratin staining in Merkel cell carcinoma: an immunohistochemical study of cytokeratins 5/6, 7, 17, and 20.**
  Author(s): Jensen K, Kohler S, Rouse RV.
  Source: Appl Immunohistochem Mol Morphol. 2000 December; 8(4): 310-5.
  http://www.ncbi.nlm.nih.gov:80/entrez/query.fcgi?cmd=Retrieve&db=PubMed&list_uids=11127923&dopt=Abstract

- **Cytomorphologic features of Merkel cell carcinoma in fine needle aspiration biopsies. A study of two atypical cases.**
  Author(s): Hallman JR, Shaw JA, Geisinger KR, Loggie BW, White WL.
  Source: Acta Cytol. 2000 March-April; 44(2): 185-93.
  http://www.ncbi.nlm.nih.gov:80/entrez/query.fcgi?cmd=Retrieve&db=PubMed&list_uids=10740605&dopt=Abstract

- **Deletion mapping of the short arm of chromosome 3 in Merkel cell carcinoma.**
  Author(s): Leonard JH, Williams G, Walters MK, Nancarrow DJ, Rabbitts PH.
  Source: Genes, Chromosomes & Cancer. 1996 February; 15(2): 102-7.
  http://www.ncbi.nlm.nih.gov:80/entrez/query.fcgi?cmd=Retrieve&db=PubMed&list_uids=8834173&dopt=Abstract

- **Deletion mapping on the short arm of chromosome 1 in Merkel cell carcinoma.**
  Author(s): Leonard JH, Cook AL, Nancarrow D, Hayward N, Van Gele M, Van Roy N, Speleman F.

Source: Cancer Detection and Prevention. 2000; 24(6): 620-7.
http://www.ncbi.nlm.nih.gov:80/entrez/query.fcgi?cmd=Retrieve&db=PubMed&list_uids=11198276&dopt=Abstract

- **Deletion of chromosome arm 1p in a Merkel cell carcinoma (MCC).**
  Author(s): Gibas Z, Weil S, Chen ST, McCue PA.
  Source: Genes, Chromosomes & Cancer. 1994 March; 9(3): 216-20. Review.
  http://www.ncbi.nlm.nih.gov:80/entrez/query.fcgi?cmd=Retrieve&db=PubMed&list_uids=7515664&dopt=Abstract

- **Diagnostic pitfalls of Merkel cell carcinoma and dramatic response to chemotherapy.**
  Author(s): Chang SF, Suh JW, Choi JH, Yoon GS, Huh J, Sung KJ, Moon KC, Kim WG, Koh JK.
  Source: J Dermatol. 1998 May; 25(5): 322-8.
  http://www.ncbi.nlm.nih.gov:80/entrez/query.fcgi?cmd=Retrieve&db=PubMed&list_uids=9640886&dopt=Abstract

- **Diagnostic relevance of chromosomal in-situ hybridization in Merkel cell carcinoma: targeted interphase cytogenetic tumour analyses.**
  Author(s): Amo-Takyi BK, Tietze L, Tory K, Guerreiro P, Gunther K, Bhardwaj RS, Mittermayer C, Handt S.
  Source: Histopathology. 1999 February; 34(2): 163-9.
  http://www.ncbi.nlm.nih.gov:80/entrez/query.fcgi?cmd=Retrieve&db=PubMed&list_uids=10064396&dopt=Abstract

- **Differences of bcl-2 protein expression between Merkel cells and Merkel cell carcinomas.**
  Author(s): Moll I, Gillardon F, Waltering S, Schmelz M, Moll R.
  Source: Journal of Cutaneous Pathology. 1996 April; 23(2): 109-17.
  http://www.ncbi.nlm.nih.gov:80/entrez/query.fcgi?cmd=Retrieve&db=PubMed&list_uids=8721444&dopt=Abstract

- **Differentiation between merkel cell carcinoma and malignant melanoma: An immunohistochemical study.**
  Author(s): Kontochristopoulos GJ, Stavropoulos PG, Krasagakis K, Goerdt S, Zouboulis CC.
  Source: Dermatology (Basel, Switzerland). 2000; 201(2): 123-6.
  http://www.ncbi.nlm.nih.gov:80/entrez/query.fcgi?cmd=Retrieve&db=PubMed&list_uids=11053914&dopt=Abstract

- **Early aggressive treatment for Merkel cell carcinoma improves outcome.**
  Author(s): Kokoska ER, Kokoska MS, Collins BT, Stapleton DR, Wade TP.
  Source: American Journal of Surgery. 1997 December; 174(6): 688-93.
  http://www.ncbi.nlm.nih.gov:80/entrez/query.fcgi?cmd=Retrieve&db=PubMed&list_uids=9409598&dopt=Abstract

- **Early experience with sentinel lymph node mapping for Merkel cell carcinoma.**
  Author(s): Rodrigues LK, Leong SP, Kashani-Sabet M, Wong JH.
  Source: Journal of the American Academy of Dermatology. 2001 August; 45(2): 303-8.
  http://www.ncbi.nlm.nih.gov:80/entrez/query.fcgi?cmd=Retrieve&db=PubMed&list_uids=11464197&dopt=Abstract

- **Erythematous nodule on a woman's face. Diagnosis: Merkel cell carcinoma.**
  Author(s): Juzych LA, Nordby CA.
  Source: Archives of Dermatology. 2001 October; 137(10): 1367-72. No Abstract Available.
  http://www.ncbi.nlm.nih.gov:80/entrez/query.fcgi?cmd=Retrieve&db=PubMed&list_uids=11594867&dopt=Abstract

- **Expression of alpha subunit of guanine nucleotide-binding protein Go in Merkel cell carcinoma.**
  Author(s): Uhara H, Wang YL, Matsumoto S, Kawachi S, Saida T.
  Source: Journal of Cutaneous Pathology. 1995 April; 22(2): 146-8.
  http://www.ncbi.nlm.nih.gov:80/entrez/query.fcgi?cmd=Retrieve&db=PubMed&list_uids=7560347&dopt=Abstract

- **Expression of bcl-2 and p53 in Merkel cell carcinoma. An immunohistochemical study.**
  Author(s): Kennedy MM, Blessing K, King G, Kerr KM.
  Source: The American Journal of Dermatopathology. 1996 June; 18(3): 273-7.
  http://www.ncbi.nlm.nih.gov:80/entrez/query.fcgi?cmd=Retrieve&db=PubMed&list_uids=8806961&dopt=Abstract

- **Expression of the apoptosis-related oncogenes bcl-2, bax, and p53 in Merkel cell carcinoma: can they predict treatment response and clinical outcome?**

Author(s): Feinmesser M, Halpern M, Fenig E, Tsabari C, Hodak E, Sulkes J, Brenner B, Okon E.
Source: Human Pathology. 1999 November; 30(11): 1367-72.
http://www.ncbi.nlm.nih.gov:80/entrez/query.fcgi?cmd=Retrieve&db=PubMed&list_uids=10571519&dopt=Abstract

- **Farnesylthiosalicylic acid inhibits the growth of human Merkel cell carcinoma in SCID mice.**
  Author(s): Jansen B, Heere-Ress E, Schlagbauer-Wadl H, Halaschek-Wiener J, Waltering S, Moll I, Pehamberger H, Marciano D, Kloog Y, Wolff K.
  Source: Journal of Molecular Medicine (Berlin, Germany). 1999 November; 77(11): 792-7.
  http://www.ncbi.nlm.nih.gov:80/entrez/query.fcgi?cmd=Retrieve&db=PubMed&list_uids=10619439&dopt=Abstract

- **Fine-needle aspiration of Merkel cell carcinoma of the skin with cytomorphology and immunocytochemical correlation.**
  Author(s): Collins BT, Elmberger PG, Tani EM, Bjornhagen V, Ramos RR.
  Source: Diagnostic Cytopathology. 1998 April; 18(4): 251-7.
  http://www.ncbi.nlm.nih.gov:80/entrez/query.fcgi?cmd=Retrieve&db=PubMed&list_uids=9557258&dopt=Abstract

- **Frequent allelic loss at 10q23 but low incidence of PTEN mutations in Merkel cell carcinoma.**
  Author(s): Van Gele M, Leonard JH, Van Roy N, Cook AL, De Paepe A, Speleman F.
  Source: International Journal of Cancer. Journal International Du Cancer. 2001 May 1; 92(3): 409-13.
  http://www.ncbi.nlm.nih.gov:80/entrez/query.fcgi?cmd=Retrieve&db=PubMed&list_uids=11291079&dopt=Abstract

- **Ga-67 citrate scintigraphy in Merkel cell carcinoma.**
  Author(s): Wakisaka M, Miyake H, Sai M, Takeoka H, Mori H, Anzai S, Okamoto O, Takayasu S.
  Source: Clinical Nuclear Medicine. 1998 November; 23(11): 787-9. No Abstract Available.
  http://www.ncbi.nlm.nih.gov:80/entrez/query.fcgi?cmd=Retrieve&db=PubMed&list_uids=9814578&dopt=Abstract

- **Genetic changes associated with primary Merkel cell carcinoma.**
  Author(s): Vortmeyer AO, Merino MJ, Boni R, Liotta LA, Cavazzana A, Zhuang Z.
  Source: Am J Clin Pathol. 1998 May; 109(5): 565-70.
  http://www.ncbi.nlm.nih.gov:80/entrez/query.fcgi?cmd=Retrieve&db=PubMed&list_uids=9576574&dopt=Abstract

- **Giant Merkel cell carcinoma involving the upper extremity.**
  Author(s): Hapcic K, Panchal J, Stewart J, Levine N.
  Source: Dermatologic Surgery : Official Publication for American Society for Dermatologic Surgery [et Al.]. 2001 May; 27(5): 493-4.
  http://www.ncbi.nlm.nih.gov:80/entrez/query.fcgi?cmd=Retrieve&db=PubMed&list_uids=11359501&dopt=Abstract

- **Gingival metastasis of merkel cell carcinoma: a case report.**
  Author(s): Schmidt-Westhausen A, Reichart PA, Gross UM.
  Source: Journal of Oral Pathology & Medicine : Official Publication of the International Association of Oral Pathologists and the American Academy of Oral Pathology. 1996 January; 25(1): 44-7.
  http://www.ncbi.nlm.nih.gov:80/entrez/query.fcgi?cmd=Retrieve&db=PubMed&list_uids=8850357&dopt=Abstract

- **Growth and characterization of a cell line from a human primary neuroendocrine carcinoma of the skin (Merkel cell carcinoma) in culture and as xenograft.**
  Author(s): Krasagakis K, Almond-Roesler B, Geilen C, Fimmel S, Krengel S, Chatzaki E, Gravanis A, Orfanos CE.
  Source: Journal of Cellular Physiology. 2001 June; 187(3): 386-91.
  http://www.ncbi.nlm.nih.gov:80/entrez/query.fcgi?cmd=Retrieve&db=PubMed&list_uids=11319762&dopt=Abstract

- **Guess What! Cutaneous Merkel cell carcinoma of the left lower leg.**
  Author(s): Stone N, Burge S.
  Source: Eur J Dermatol. 1998 June; 8(4): 285-6. No Abstract Available.
  http://www.ncbi.nlm.nih.gov:80/entrez/query.fcgi?cmd=Retrieve&db=PubMed&list_uids=9917174&dopt=Abstract

- **Imaging of Merkel cell carcinoma.**
  Author(s): Nguyen BD, McCullough AE.

Source: Radiographics : a Review Publication of the Radiological Society of North America, Inc. 2002 March-April; 22(2): 367-76. Review.
http://www.ncbi.nlm.nih.gov:80/entrez/query.fcgi?cmd=Retrieve&db= PubMed&list_uids=11896226&dopt=Abstract

- **Immunohistochemical analysis of sentinel lymph nodes from patients with Merkel cell carcinoma.**
  Author(s): Allen PJ, Busam K, Hill AD, Stojadinovic A, Coit DG.
  Source: Cancer. 2001 September 15; 92(6): 1650-5.
  http://www.ncbi.nlm.nih.gov:80/entrez/query.fcgi?cmd=Retrieve&db= PubMed&list_uids=11745244&dopt=Abstract

- **Immunohistochemical and immunoelectron microscopic demonstration of chromogranin A in formalin-fixed tissue of Merkel cell carcinoma.**
  Author(s): Haneke E, Schulze HJ, Mahrle G.
  Source: Journal of the American Academy of Dermatology. 1993 February; 28(2 Pt 1): 222-6.
  http://www.ncbi.nlm.nih.gov:80/entrez/query.fcgi?cmd=Retrieve&db= PubMed&list_uids=8432919&dopt=Abstract

- **Immunohistochemical detection of cathepsins in Merkel cell carcinomas.**
  Author(s): Thewes M, Engst R, Ring J.
  Source: Acta Dermato-Venereologica. 1997 July; 77(4): 328-9. No Abstract Available.
  http://www.ncbi.nlm.nih.gov:80/entrez/query.fcgi?cmd=Retrieve&db= PubMed&list_uids=9228235&dopt=Abstract

- **Immunohistochemical studies of Merkel cell carcinoma of the eyelid.**
  Author(s): Furuno K, Wakakura M, Shimizu K, Iwabuchi K, Kameya T.
  Source: Japanese Journal of Ophthalmology. 1992; 36(3): 348-55.
  http://www.ncbi.nlm.nih.gov:80/entrez/query.fcgi?cmd=Retrieve&db= PubMed&list_uids=1281512&dopt=Abstract

- **Immunostaining for cytokeratin 20 improves detection of micrometastatic Merkel cell carcinoma in sentinel lymph nodes.**
  Author(s): Su LD, Lowe L, Bradford CR, Yahanda AI, Johnson TM, Sondak VK.

Source: Journal of the American Academy of Dermatology. 2002 May; 46(5): 661-6.

http://www.ncbi.nlm.nih.gov:80/entrez/query.fcgi?cmd=Retrieve&db=PubMed&list_uids=12004304&dopt=Abstract

- **Immunostaining for thyroid transcription factor 1 and cytokeratin 20 aids the distinction of small cell carcinoma from Merkel cell carcinoma, but not pulmonary from extrapulmonary small cell carcinomas.**
  Author(s): Cheuk W, Kwan MY, Suster S, Chan JK.
  Source: Archives of Pathology & Laboratory Medicine. 2001 February; 125(2): 228-31.

  http://www.ncbi.nlm.nih.gov:80/entrez/query.fcgi?cmd=Retrieve&db=PubMed&list_uids=11175640&dopt=Abstract

- **Indium-111 octreotide scintigraphy of Merkel cell carcinomas and their metastases.**
  Author(s): Guitera-Rovel P, Lumbroso J, Gautier-Gougis MS, Spatz A, Mercier S, Margulis A, Mamelle G, Kolb F, Lartigau E, Avril MF.
  Source: Annals of Oncology : Official Journal of the European Society for Medical Oncology / Esmo. 2001 June; 12(6): 807-11.

  http://www.ncbi.nlm.nih.gov:80/entrez/query.fcgi?cmd=Retrieve&db=PubMed&list_uids=11484956&dopt=Abstract

- **Insights into the Merkel cell phenotype from Merkel cell carcinoma cell lines.**
  Author(s): Leonard JH, Bell JR.
  Source: The Australasian Journal of Dermatology. 1997 June; 38 Suppl 1: S91-8. Review.

  http://www.ncbi.nlm.nih.gov:80/entrez/query.fcgi?cmd=Retrieve&db=PubMed&list_uids=10994482&dopt=Abstract

- **Intraepidermal Merkel cell carcinoma with no dermal involvement.**
  Author(s): Brown HA, Sawyer DM, Woo T.
  Source: The American Journal of Dermatopathology. 2000 February; 22(1): 65-9.

  http://www.ncbi.nlm.nih.gov:80/entrez/query.fcgi?cmd=Retrieve&db=PubMed&list_uids=10698220&dopt=Abstract

- **Intraoperative lymphatic mapping and sentinel lymph node biopsy for Merkel cell carcinoma.**
  Author(s): Hill AD, Brady MS, Coit DG.

Source: The British Journal of Surgery. 1999 April; 86(4): 518-21.
http://www.ncbi.nlm.nih.gov:80/entrez/query.fcgi?cmd=Retrieve&db=PubMed&list_uids=10215828&dopt=Abstract

- **Is aggressive surgical management justified in the treatment of Merkel cell carcinoma?**
  Author(s): Shack RB, Barton RM, DeLozier J, Rees RS, Lynch JB.
  Source: Plastic and Reconstructive Surgery. 1994 December; 94(7): 970-5.
  http://www.ncbi.nlm.nih.gov:80/entrez/query.fcgi?cmd=Retrieve&db=PubMed&list_uids=7661915&dopt=Abstract

- **Is there a diminishing role for surgery for Merkel cell carcinoma of the skin? a review of current management.**
  Author(s): Poulsen M, Harvey J.
  Source: Anz Journal of Surgery. 2002 February; 72(2): 142-6. Review.
  http://www.ncbi.nlm.nih.gov:80/entrez/query.fcgi?cmd=Retrieve&db=PubMed&list_uids=12074067&dopt=Abstract

- **Keratin 20: immunohistochemical marker for gastrointestinal, urothelial, and Merkel cell carcinomas.**
  Author(s): Miettinen M.
  Source: Modern Pathology : an Official Journal of the United States and Canadian Academy of Pathology, Inc. 1995 May; 8(4): 384-8.
  http://www.ncbi.nlm.nih.gov:80/entrez/query.fcgi?cmd=Retrieve&db=PubMed&list_uids=7567935&dopt=Abstract

- **Lectin and proteoglycan histochemistry of Merkel cell carcinomas.**
  Author(s): Sames K, Schumacher U, Halata Z, Van Damme EJ, Peumans WJ, Asmus B, Moll R, Moll I.
  Source: Experimental Dermatology. 2001 April; 10(2): 100-9.
  http://www.ncbi.nlm.nih.gov:80/entrez/query.fcgi?cmd=Retrieve&db=PubMed&list_uids=11260248&dopt=Abstract

- **Loss of heterozygosity of chromosome 13 in Merkel cell carcinoma.**
  Author(s): Leonard JH, Hayard N.
  Source: Genes, Chromosomes & Cancer. 1997 September; 20(1): 93-7.
  http://www.ncbi.nlm.nih.gov:80/entrez/query.fcgi?cmd=Retrieve&db=PubMed&list_uids=9290960&dopt=Abstract

- **Lumbosacral metastatic extradural Merkel cell carcinoma causing nerve root compression--case report.**
  Author(s): Turgut M, Gokpinar D, Barutca S, Erkus M.

Source: Neurol Med Chir (Tokyo). 2002 February; 42(2): 78-80.
http://www.ncbi.nlm.nih.gov:80/entrez/query.fcgi?cmd=Retrieve&db=PubMed&list_uids=11944594&dopt=Abstract

- **Lymph node Merkel cell carcinoma with no evidence of cutaneous tumor--report of two cases.**
  Author(s): Ferrara G, Ianniello GP, Di Vizio D, Nappi O.
  Source: Tumori. 1997 September-October; 83(5): 868-72.
  http://www.ncbi.nlm.nih.gov:80/entrez/query.fcgi?cmd=Retrieve&db=PubMed&list_uids=9428924&dopt=Abstract

- **Lymphangiectomy and treatment modalities in Merkel cell carcinoma: a report of five new cases.**
  Author(s): Vandeput JJ, Kerre S, Vandepitte J, Janssens J.
  Source: Anticancer Res. 1996 November-December; 16(6B): 3887-93. Review.
  http://www.ncbi.nlm.nih.gov:80/entrez/query.fcgi?cmd=Retrieve&db=PubMed&list_uids=9042276&dopt=Abstract

- **Lymphatic mapping for Merkel cell carcinoma.**
  Author(s): Kurul S, Mudun A, Aksakal N, Aygen M.
  Source: Plastic and Reconstructive Surgery. 2000 February; 105(2): 680-3.
  http://www.ncbi.nlm.nih.gov:80/entrez/query.fcgi?cmd=Retrieve&db=PubMed&list_uids=10697177&dopt=Abstract

- **Lymphoscintigraphy with sentinel lymph node biopsy in cutaneous Merkel cell carcinoma.**
  Author(s): Sian KU, Wagner JD, Sood R, Park HM, Havlik R, Coleman JJ.
  Source: Annals of Plastic Surgery. 1999 June; 42(6): 679-82.
  http://www.ncbi.nlm.nih.gov:80/entrez/query.fcgi?cmd=Retrieve&db=PubMed&list_uids=10382808&dopt=Abstract

- **Lymphoscintigraphy, sentinel lymph node biopsy, and Mohs micrographic surgery in the treatment of Merkel cell carcinoma.**
  Author(s): Zeitouni NC, Cheney RT, Delacure MD.
  Source: Dermatologic Surgery : Official Publication for American Society for Dermatologic Surgery [et Al.]. 2000 January; 26(1): 12-8.
  http://www.ncbi.nlm.nih.gov:80/entrez/query.fcgi?cmd=Retrieve&db=PubMed&list_uids=10632680&dopt=Abstract

- **Magnetic resonance imaging appearance of metastatic Merkel cell carcinoma to the sacrum and epidural space.**
  Author(s): Moayed S, Maldjianb C, Adam R, Bonakdarpour A.
  Source: Magnetic Resonance Imaging. 2000 October; 18(8): 1039-42.
  http://www.ncbi.nlm.nih.gov:80/entrez/query.fcgi?cmd=Retrieve&db=PubMed&list_uids=11121710&dopt=Abstract

- **Malignant melanoma with clinical and histologic features of Merkel cell carcinoma.**
  Author(s): House NS, Fedok F, Maloney ME, Helm KF.
  Source: Journal of the American Academy of Dermatology. 1994 November; 31(5 Pt 2): 839-42.
  http://www.ncbi.nlm.nih.gov:80/entrez/query.fcgi?cmd=Retrieve&db=PubMed&list_uids=7525666&dopt=Abstract

- **Management and prognosis of Merkel cell carcinoma of the eyelid.**
  Author(s): Peters GB 3rd, Meyer DR, Shields JA, Custer PL, Rubin PA, Wojno TH, Bersani TA, Tanenbaum M.
  Source: Ophthalmology. 2001 September; 108(9): 1575-9.
  http://www.ncbi.nlm.nih.gov:80/entrez/query.fcgi?cmd=Retrieve&db=PubMed&list_uids=11535453&dopt=Abstract

- **Management of Merkel cell carcinoma.**
  Author(s): Plunkett TA, Subrumanian R, Leslie MD, Harper PG.
  Source: Expert Rev Anticancer Ther. 2001 October; 1(3): 441-5. Review.
  http://www.ncbi.nlm.nih.gov:80/entrez/query.fcgi?cmd=Retrieve&db=PubMed&list_uids=12113110&dopt=Abstract

- **Merkel cell carcinoma (neuroendocrine carcinoma of the skin).**
  Author(s): Smith PD, Patterson JW.
  Source: Am J Clin Pathol. 2001 June; 115 Suppl: S68-78. Review.
  http://www.ncbi.nlm.nih.gov:80/entrez/query.fcgi?cmd=Retrieve&db=PubMed&list_uids=11993692&dopt=Abstract

- **Merkel cell carcinoma and chronic arsenicism.**
  Author(s): Lien HC, Tsai TF, Lee YY, Hsiao CH.
  Source: Journal of the American Academy of Dermatology. 1999 October; 41(4): 641-3.
  http://www.ncbi.nlm.nih.gov:80/entrez/query.fcgi?cmd=Retrieve&db=PubMed&list_uids=10495389&dopt=Abstract

- **Merkel cell carcinoma and HIV infection.**
  Author(s): Engels EA, Frisch M, Goedert JJ, Biggar RJ, Miller RW.
  Source: Lancet. 2002 February 9; 359(9305): 497-8.
  http://www.ncbi.nlm.nih.gov:80/entrez/query.fcgi?cmd=Retrieve&db=PubMed&list_uids=11853800&dopt=Abstract

- **Merkel cell carcinoma and iodine-131 metaiodobenzylguanidine scan.**
  Author(s): Castagnoli A, Biti G, De Cristofaro MT, Ferri P, Magrini SM, Papi MG, Bianchi S.
  Source: European Journal of Nuclear Medicine. 1992; 19(10): 913-6.
  http://www.ncbi.nlm.nih.gov:80/entrez/query.fcgi?cmd=Retrieve&db=PubMed&list_uids=1451708&dopt=Abstract

- **Merkel cell carcinoma and melanoma: etiological similarities and differences.**
  Author(s): Miller RW, Rabkin CS.
  Source: Cancer Epidemiology, Biomarkers & Prevention : a Publication of the American Association for Cancer Research, Cosponsored by the American Society of Preventive Oncology. 1999 February; 8(2): 153-8.
  http://www.ncbi.nlm.nih.gov:80/entrez/query.fcgi?cmd=Retrieve&db=PubMed&list_uids=10067813&dopt=Abstract

- **Merkel cell carcinoma and multiple Bowen's disease: incidental association or possible relationship to inorganic arsenic exposure?**
  Author(s): Ohnishi Y, Murakami S, Ohtsuka H, Miyauchi S, Shinmori H, Hashimoto K.
  Source: J Dermatol. 1997 May; 24(5): 310-6.
  http://www.ncbi.nlm.nih.gov:80/entrez/query.fcgi?cmd=Retrieve&db=PubMed&list_uids=9198320&dopt=Abstract

Vocabulary Builder

Abdominal: Having to do with the abdomen, which is the part of the body between the chest and the hips that contains the pancreas, stomach, intestines, liver, gallbladder, and other organs. [NIH]

Apoptosis: A normal series of events in a cell that leads to its death. [NIH]

Assay: Determination of the amount of a particular constituent of a mixture, or of the biological or pharmacological potency of a drug. [EU]

Atypical: Irregular; not conformable to the type; in microbiology, applied specifically to strains of unusual type. [EU]

Biomarkers: Substances sometimes found in an increased amount in the blood, other body fluids, or tissues and that may suggest the presence of some types of cancer. Biomarkers include CA 125 (ovarian cancer), CA 15-3 (breast cancer), CEA (ovarian, lung, breast, pancreas, and GI tract cancers), and PSA (prostate cancer). Also called tumor markers. [NIH]

Carboplatin: An anticancer drug that belongs to the family of drugs called platinum compounds. [NIH]

Carcinoid: A type of tumor usually found in the gastrointestinal system (most often in the appendix), and sometimes in the lungs or other sites. Carcinoid tumors are usually benign. [NIH]

Cathepsins: A group of lysosomal proteinases or endopeptidases found in aqueous extracts of a variety of animal tissue. They function optimally within an acidic pH range. [NIH]

Chromosomal: Pertaining to chromosomes. [EU]

Chromosome: Part of a cell that contains genetic information. Except for sperm and eggs, all human cells contain 46 chromosomes. [NIH]

Chronic: A disease or condition that persists or progresses over a long period of time. [NIH]

Cytogenetics: A branch of genetics which deals with the cytological and molecular behavior of genes and chromosomes during cell division. [NIH]

Dysplasia: Cells that look abnormal under a microscope but are not cancer. [NIH]

Epidermal: Pertaining to or resembling epidermis. Called also epidermic or epidermoid. [EU]

Epidural: The space between the wall of the spinal canal and the covering of the spinal cord. An epidural injection is given into this space. [NIH]

Etoposide: An anticancer drug that is a podophyllotoxin derivative and belongs to the family of drugs called mitotic inhibitors. [NIH]

Extremity: A limb; an arm or leg (membrum); sometimes applied specifically to a hand or foot. [EU]

Gastrointestinal: Refers to the stomach and intestines. [NIH]

Hybridization: The genetic process of crossbreeding to produce a hybrid. Hybrid nucleic acids can be formed by nucleic acid hybridization of DNA and RNA molecules. Protein hybridization allows for hybrid proteins to be formed from polypeptide chains. [NIH]

Immunohistochemistry: Histochemical localization of immunoreactive substances using labeled antibodies as reagents. [NIH]

Immunology: The study of the body's immune system. [NIH]

Incidental: 1. small and relatively unimportant, minor; 2. accompanying, but not a major part of something; 3. (to something) liable to occur because of something or in connection with something (said of risks, responsibilities, ...) [EU]

Innervation: 1. the distribution or supply of nerves to a part. 2. the supply of nervous energy or of nerve stimulus sent to a part. [EU]

Interphase: The interval between two successive cell divisions during which the chromosomes are not individually distinguishable and DNA replication occurs. [NIH]

Iodine: A nonmetallic element of the halogen group that is represented by the atomic symbol I, atomic number 53, and atomic weight of 126.90. It is a nutritionally essential element, especially important in thyroid hormone synthesis. In solution, it has anti-infective properties and is used topically. [NIH]

Mechanoreceptors: Cells specialized to transduce mechanical stimuli and relay that information centrally in the nervous system. Mechanoreceptors include hair cells, which mediate hearing and balance, and the various somatosensory receptors, often with non-neural accessory structures. [NIH]

Melanocytes: Cells in the skin that produce and contain the pigment called melanin. [NIH]

Metastasis: The spread of cancer from one part of the body to another. Tumors formed from cells that have spread are called "secondary tumors" and contain cells that are like those in the original (primary) tumor. The plural is metastases. [NIH]

Neural: 1. pertaining to a nerve or to the nerves. 2. situated in the region of the spinal axis, as the neutral arch. [EU]

Neurology: A medical specialty concerned with the study of the structures, functions, and diseases of the nervous system. [NIH]

Neurons: The basic cellular units of nervous tissue. Each neuron consists of a body, an axon, and dendrites. Their purpose is to receive, conduct, and transmit impulses in the nervous system. [NIH]

Octreotide: A drug similar to the naturally occurring growth hormone inhibitor somatostatin. Octreotide is used to treat diarrhea and flushing associated with certain types of tumors. [NIH]

Oncogene: A gene that normally directs cell growth. If altered, an oncogene can promote or allow the uncontrolled growth of cancer. Alterations can be inherited or caused by an environmental exposure to carcinogens. [NIH]

Ophthalmology: A surgical specialty concerned with the structure and function of the eye and the medical and surgical treatment of its defects and diseases. [NIH]

Oral: By or having to do with the mouth. [NIH]

Orbital: Pertaining to the orbit (= the bony cavity that contains the eyeball). [EU]

Otolaryngology: A surgical specialty concerned with the study and treatment of disorders of the ear, nose, and throat. [NIH]

Pancreas: A glandular organ located in the abdomen. It makes pancreatic juices, which contain enzymes that aid in digestion, and it produces several hormones, including insulin. The pancreas is surrounded by the stomach, intestines, and other organs. [NIH]

Pathologist: A doctor who identifies diseases by studying cells and tissues under a microscope. [NIH]

Perinatal: Pertaining to or occurring in the period shortly before and after birth; variously defined as beginning with completion of the twentieth to twenty-eighth week of gestation and ending 7 to 28 days after birth. [EU]

Precursor: Something that precedes. In biological processes, a substance from which another, usually more active or mature substance is formed. In clinical medicine, a sign or symptom that heralds another. [EU]

Proteins: Polymers of amino acids linked by peptide bonds. The specific sequence of amino acids determines the shape and function of the protein. [NIH]

Proteoglycan: A molecule that contains both protein and glycosaminoglycans, which are a type of polysaccharide. Proteoglycans are found in cartilage and other connective tissues. [NIH]

Pulmonary: Relating to the lungs. [NIH]

Radiology: The use of radiation (such as x-rays) or other imaging technologies (such as ultrasound and magnetic resonance imaging) to diagnose or treat disease. [NIH]

Radium: Radium. A radioactive element of the alkaline earth series of metals. It has the atomic symbol Ra, atomic number 88, and atomic weight 226. Radium is the product of the disintegration of uranium and is present in pitchblende and all ores containing uranium. It is used clinically as a source of beta and gamma-rays in radiotherapy, particularly brachytherapy. [NIH]

Relapse: The return of signs and symptoms of cancer after a period of improvement. [NIH]

Tomography: A series of detailed pictures of areas inside the body; the pictures are created by a computer linked to an x-ray machine. [NIH]

Toxicity: The quality of being poisonous, especially the degree of virulence of a toxic microbe or of a poison. [EU]

Trisomy: The possession of a third chromosome of any one type in an otherwise diploid cell. [NIH]

Tumour: 1. swelling, one of the cardinal signs of inflammations; morbid enlargement. 2. a new growth of tissue in which the multiplication of cells is uncontrolled and progressive; called also neoplasm. [EU]

Vitiligo: A disorder consisting of areas of macular depigmentation, commonly on extensor aspects of extremities, on the face or neck, and in skin folds. Age of onset is often in young adulthood and the condition tends to progress gradually with lesions enlarging and extending until a quiescent state is reached. [NIH]

Xenograft: The cells of one species transplanted to another species. [NIH]

CHAPTER 5. BOOKS ON MERKEL CELL CARCINOMA

Overview

This chapter provides bibliographic book references relating to merkel cell carcinoma. You have many options to locate books on merkel cell carcinoma. The simplest method is to go to your local bookseller and inquire about titles that they have in stock or can special order for you. Some patients, however, feel uncomfortable approaching their local booksellers and prefer online sources (e.g. www.amazon.com and www.bn.com). In addition to online booksellers, excellent sources for book titles on merkel cell carcinoma include the Combined Health Information Database and the National Library of Medicine. Once you have found a title that interests you, visit your local public or medical library to see if it is available for loan.

The National Library of Medicine Book Index

The National Library of Medicine at the National Institutes of Health has a massive database of books published on healthcare and biomedicine. Go to the following Internet site, **http://locatorplus.gov/**, and then select "Search LOCATORplus." Once you are in the search area, simply type "merkel cell carcinoma" (or synonyms) into the search box, and select "books only." From there, results can be sorted by publication date, author, or relevance. The following was recently catalogued by the National Library of Medicine:[30]

---

[30] In addition to LOCATORPlus, in collaboration with authors and publishers, the National Center for Biotechnology Information (NCBI) is adapting biomedical books for the Web. The books may be accessed in two ways: (1) by searching directly using any search term or phrase (in the same way as the bibliographic database PubMed), or (2) by following the

- **Merkel cells, Merkel cell carcinoma, and neurobiology of the skin: proceedings of the 1st Symposium of the Japanese Society for Ultrastructural Cutaneous Biology held in Tokyo, Japan, 24-25 November 1999.** Author: editors, Hiroyuki Suzuki, Tomomichi Ono; Year: 2000; Amsterdam; New York: Elsevier, 2000. ; ISBN: 0444502211
http://www.amazon.com/exec/obidos/ASIN/0444502211/icongroupinterna

Chapters on Merkel Cell Carcinoma

Frequently, merkel cell carcinoma will be discussed within a book, perhaps within a specific chapter. In order to find chapters that are specifically dealing with merkel cell carcinoma, an excellent source of abstracts is the Combined Health Information Database. You will need to limit your search to book chapters and merkel cell carcinoma using the "Detailed Search" option. Go directly to the following hyperlink: **http://chid.nih.gov/detail/detail.html**. To find book chapters, use the drop boxes at the bottom of the search page where "You may refine your search by." Select the dates and language you prefer, and the format option "Book Chapter." By making these selections and typing in "merkel cell carcinoma" (or synonyms) into the "For these words:" box, you will only receive results on chapters in books.

General Home References

In addition to references for merkel cell carcinoma, you may want a general home medical guide that spans all aspects of home healthcare. The following list is a recent sample of such guides (sorted alphabetically by title; hyperlinks provide rankings, information, and reviews at Amazon.com):

- **Cancer: 50 Essential Things to Do** by Greg Anderson, O. Carl Simonton; Paperback - 184 pages; Revised & Updated edition (August 1999), Plume; ISBN: 0452280745;
http://www.amazon.com/exec/obidos/ASIN/0452280745/icongroupinterna

---

links to PubMed abstracts. Each PubMed abstract has a "Books" button that displays a facsimile of the abstract in which some phrases are hypertext links. These phrases are also found in the books available at NCBI. Click on hyperlinked results in the list of books in which the phrase is found. Currently, the majority of the links are between the books and PubMed. In the future, more links will be created between the books and other types of information, such as gene and protein sequences and macromolecular structures. See **http://www.ncbi.nlm.nih.gov/entrez/query.fcgi?db=Books.**

- **Cancer Encyclopedia -- Collections of Anti-Cancer & Anti-Carcinogenic Agents, Chemicals, Drugs and Substances** by John C. Bartone; Paperback (January 2002), ABBE Publishers Association of Washington, DC; ISBN: 0788326791;
  http://www.amazon.com/exec/obidos/ASIN/0788326791/icongroupinterna

- **Cancer Sourcebook: Basic Consumer Health Information About Major Forms and Stages of Cancer** by Edward J. Prucha (Editor); Library Binding - 1100 pages, 3rd edition (August 1, 2000), Omnigraphics, Inc.; ISBN: 0780802276;
  http://www.amazon.com/exec/obidos/ASIN/0780802276/icongroupinterna

- **Cancer Supportive Care: A Comprehensive Guide for Patients and Their Families** by Ernest H. Rosenbaum, M.D., Isadora Rosenbaum, M.A.; Paperback - 472 pages (November 5, 1998), Somerville House Books Limited; ISBN: 1894042115;
  http://www.amazon.com/exec/obidos/ASIN/1894042115/icongroupinterna

- **Cancer Symptom Management: Patient Self-Care Guides (Book with CD-ROM for Windows & Macintosh)** by Connie Henke Yarbro (Editor), et al; CD-ROM - 264 pages, 2nd Book & CD-Rom edition (January 15, 2000), Jones & Bartlett Publishing; ISBN: 0763711675;
  http://www.amazon.com/exec/obidos/ASIN/0763711675/icongroupinterna

- **Diagnosis Cancer: Your Guide Through the First Few Months** by Wendy Schlessel Harpham, Ann Bliss Pilcher (Illustrator); Paperback: 230 pages; Revised & Updated edition (November 1997), .W. Norton & Company; ISBN: 0393316912;
  http://www.amazon.com/exec/obidos/ASIN/0393316912/icongroupinterna

- **The Human Side of Cancer: Living with Hope, Coping with Uncertainty** by Jimmie C. Holland, M.D., Sheldon Lewis; Paperback - 368 pages (October 2, 2001), Quill; ISBN: 006093042X;
  http://www.amazon.com/exec/obidos/ASIN/006093042X/icongroupinterna

Vocabulary Builder

Anus: The opening of the rectum to the outside of the body. [NIH]

Auditory: Pertaining to the sense of hearing. [EU]

Carcinogenic: Producing carcinoma. [EU]

Cervix: The lower, narrow end of the uterus that forms a canal between the uterus and vagina. [NIH]

Chloroquine: The prototypical antimalarial agent with a mechanism that is not well understood. It has also been used to treat rheumatoid arthritis, systemic lupus erythematosus, and in the systemic therapy of amebic liver abscesses. [NIH]

Esophagus: The muscular tube through which food passes from the throat to the stomach. [NIH]

Larynx: The area of the throat containing the vocal cords and used for breathing, swallowing, and talking. Also called the voice box. [NIH]

Membrane: A very thin layer of tissue that covers a surface. [NIH]

Mucosa: A mucous membrane, or tunica mucosa. [EU]

Nasopharynx: The upper part of the throat behind the nose. An opening on each side of the nasopharynx leads into the ear. [NIH]

Occult: Obscure; concealed from observation, difficult to understand. [EU]

Palate: The roof of the mouth. The front portion is bony (hard palate), and the back portion is muscular (soft palate). [NIH]

Rectum: The last 8 to 10 inches of the large intestine. [NIH]

Skeletal: Having to do with the skeleton (boney part of the body). [NIH]

Virus: Submicroscopic organism that causes infectious disease. In cancer therapy, some viruses may be made into vaccines that help the body build an immune response to, and kill, tumor cells. [NIH]

Vulva: The external female genital organs, including the clitoris, vaginal lips, and the opening to the vagina. [NIH]

CHAPTER 6. PHYSICIAN GUIDELINES AND DATABASES

Overview

Doctors and medical researchers rely on a number of information sources to help patients with their conditions. Many will subscribe to journals or newsletters published by their professional associations or refer to specialized textbooks or clinical guides published for the medical profession. In this chapter, we focus on databases and Internet-based guidelines created or written for this professional audience.

NIH Guidelines

For the more common diseases, The National Institutes of Health publish guidelines that are frequently consulted by physicians. Publications are typically written by one or more of the various NIH Institutes. For physician guidelines, commonly referred to as "clinical" or "professional" guidelines, you can visit the following Institutes:

- Office of the Director (OD); guidelines consolidated across agencies available at **http://www.nih.gov/health/consumer/conkey.htm**

- National Institute of General Medical Sciences (NIGMS); fact sheets available at **http://www.nigms.nih.gov/news/facts/**

- National Library of Medicine (NLM); extensive encyclopedia (A.D.A.M., Inc.) with guidelines:
  http://www.nlm.nih.gov/medlineplus/healthtopics.html

- National Cancer Institute (NCI); guidelines available at
  http://cancernet.nci.nih.gov/pdq/pdq_treatment.shtml

In this chapter, we begin by reproducing one such guideline for merkel cell carcinoma:

What Is Merkel Cell Carcinoma?[31]

Merkel cell carcinoma (MCC), or neuroendocrine carcinoma of the skin, is an uncommon and often aggressive malignancy that has a poor prognosis. The Merkel cell is located in or near the basal layer of the epidermis and is closely associated with terminal axons.[32] MCC is predominantly a tumor of the elderly, and most reported cases have occurred in Caucasians.[33] It occurs most frequently in the head and neck region and in the extremities, and has a predilection for the periocular region.[34] While MCC may be difficult to diagnose, it usually presents as a painless, indurated, solitary dermal nodule with a slightly erythematous to deeply violaceous color. MCC frequently involves regional lymph nodes (10%-45% at initial presentation),[35] and

---

[31] The following guidelines appeared on the NCI Web site on Aug. 26, 2002. The text was last modified in May 2001. The text has been adapted for this sourcebook.

[32] Haag ML, Glass LF, Fenske NA: Merkel cell carcinoma. Diagnosis and treatment. Dermatologic Surgery 21(8): 669-683, 1995.
Ratner D, Nelson BR, Brown MD, et al.: Merkel cell carcinoma. Journal of the American Academy of Dermatology 29(2 part 1): 143-156, 1993.
Gould VE, Moll R, Moll I, et al.: Neuroendocrine (Merkel) cells of the skin: hyperplasias, dysplasias, and neoplasms. Laboratory Investigation 52(4): 334-353, 1985.

[33] Haag ML, Glass LF, Fenske NA: Merkel cell carcinoma. Diagnosis and treatment. Dermatologic Surgery 21(8): 669-683, 1995.
Ratner D, Nelson BR, Brown MD, et al.: Merkel cell carcinoma. Journal of the American Academy of Dermatology 29(2 part 1): 143-156, 1993.
Yiengpruksawan A, Coit DG, Thaler HT, et al.: Merkel cell carcinoma. Prognosis and management. Archives of Surgery 126(12): 1514-1519, 1991.
Goepfert H, Remmler D, Silva E, et al.: Merkel cell carcinoma (endocrine carcinoma of the skin) of the head and neck. Archives of Otolaryngology, Head and Neck Surgery 110(11): 707-712, 1984.
Gollard R, Weber R, Kosty MP, et al.: Merkel cell carcinoma. Review of 22 cases with surgical, pathologic, and therapeutic considerations. Cancer 88(8): 1842-1851, 2000.

[34] Haag ML, Glass LF, Fenske NA: Merkel cell carcinoma. Diagnosis and treatment. Dermatologic Surgery 21(8): 669-683, 1995.
Ratner D, Nelson BR, Brown MD, et al.: Merkel cell carcinoma. Journal of the American Academy of Dermatology 29(2 part 1): 143-156, 1993.
Goepfert H, Remmler D, Silva E, et al.: Merkel cell carcinoma (endocrine carcinoma of the skin) of the head and neck. Archives of Otolaryngology, Head and Neck Surgery 110(11): 707-712, 1984.
Gollard R, Weber R, Kosty MP, et al.: Merkel cell carcinoma. Review of 22 cases with surgical, pathologic, and therapeutic considerations. Cancer 88(8): 1842-1851, 2000.

[35] Haag ML, Glass LF, Fenske NA: Merkel cell carcinoma. Diagnosis and treatment. Dermatologic Surgery 21(8): 669-683, 1995.

between 50% and 75% of patients will develop regional lymph node metastases at some time during the course of their disease.[36] Distant metastases eventually occur in up to one half of patients, with lymph nodes, the liver, bone, brain, lung, and skin as the most common sites of distant involvement.[37] MCC can often develop an aggressive course, similar to aggressive melanoma. After excision of the primary tumor, local recurrence develops in 25% to 44% of patients, and is often associated with inadequate surgical margins.[38]

Cellular Classification

MCC is usually found within the dermis, but may extend into the subcutaneous tissue. The combination of vesicular nuclei with small nucleoli,

---

Ratner D, Nelson BR, Brown MD, et al.: Merkel cell carcinoma. Journal of the American Academy of Dermatology 29(2 part 1): 143-156, 1993.

Yiengpruksawan A, Coit DG, Thaler HT, et al.: Merkel cell carcinoma. Prognosis and management. Archives of Surgery 126(12): 1514-1519, 1991.

Goepfert H, Remmler D, Silva E, et al.: Merkel cell carcinoma (endocrine carcinoma of the skin) of the head and neck. Archives of Otolaryngology, Head and Neck Surgery 110(11): 707-712, 1984.

Tai PT, Yu E, Winquist E, et al.: Chemotherapy in neuroendocrine/Merkel cell carcinoma of the skin: case series and review of 204 cases. Journal of Clinical Oncology 18(12): 2493-2499, 2000.

[36] Haag ML, Glass LF, Fenske NA: Merkel cell carcinoma. Diagnosis and treatment. Dermatologic Surgery 21(8): 669-683, 1995.

Ratner D, Nelson BR, Brown MD, et al.: Merkel cell carcinoma. Journal of the American Academy of Dermatology 29(2 part 1): 143-156, 1993.

Yiengpruksawan A, Coit DG, Thaler HT, et al.: Merkel cell carcinoma. Prognosis and management. Archives of Surgery 126(12): 1514-1519, 1991.

[37] Haag ML, Glass LF, Fenske NA: Merkel cell carcinoma. Diagnosis and treatment. Dermatologic Surgery 21(8): 669-683, 1995.

Ratner D, Nelson BR, Brown MD, et al.: Merkel cell carcinoma. Journal of the American Academy of Dermatology 29(2 part 1): 143-156, 1993.

Goepfert H, Remmler D, Silva E, et al.: Merkel cell carcinoma (endocrine carcinoma of the skin) of the head and neck. Archives of Otolaryngology, Head and Neck Surgery 110(11): 707-712, 1984.

Gollard R, Weber R, Kosty MP, et al.: Merkel cell carcinoma. Review of 22 cases with surgical, pathologic, and therapeutic considerations. Cancer 88(8): 1842-1851, 2000.

Marks ME, Kim RY, Salter MM: Radiotherapy as an adjunct in the management of Merkel cell carcinoma. Cancer 65(1): 60-64, 1990.

[38] Haag ML, Glass LF, Fenske NA: Merkel cell carcinoma. Diagnosis and treatment. Dermatologic Surgery 21(8): 669-683, 1995.

Yiengpruksawan A, Coit DG, Thaler HT, et al.: Merkel cell carcinoma. Prognosis and management. Archives of Surgery 126(12): 1514-1519, 1991.

Goepfert H, Remmler D, Silva E, et al.: Merkel cell carcinoma (endocrine carcinoma of the skin) of the head and neck. Archives of Otolaryngology, Head and Neck Surgery 110(11): 707-712, 1984.

abundant mitoses, and apoptosis is considered to be characteristic of this tumor when evaluated within the context of certain architectural features. Histologically, MCC has been classified into three distinct subtypes:[39]

- Trabecular - cells are arranged in distinctly organoid clusters and trabeculae with occasional ribbons; individual cells are round to polygonal in shape and are compactly arranged; the tumor cell cytoplasm is comparatively abundant and often well defined; mitoses are few to moderate in number; this type of tumor is usually found adjacent to adnexal structures, particularly hair follicles; it is the least frequent histologic pattern identified.

- Intermediate - exhibits a solid and diffuse growth pattern; cells are less compactly arranged and the cytoplasm is less abundant than in the trabecular type; mitoses and focal areas of necrosis are frequently seen; these tumors also arise adjacent to adnexa, but may invade the epidermis; this is the most frequent histologic subtype identified; and tumors of this type may behave in a clinically more aggressive manner than those of the trabecular type.

- Small cell type - closely mimics small cell tumors of other sites; the tumors arise in the dermis and appear as solid sheets and clusters of cells; areas of necrosis and "crushing" artifact are frequently seen; the clinical behavior of this subtype appears to be as aggressive as that of the intermediate subtype.

Stage Information

There is no widely accepted or standardized staging classification based upon prognosis. A staging system based upon clinical presentation is as follows:[40]

- Stage I: Primary tumor, with no evidence of spread to lymph nodes or distant sites.

- Stage II: Regional node involvement, but no evidence of distant metastases.

---

[39] Haag ML, Glass LF, Fenske NA: Merkel cell carcinoma. Diagnosis and treatment. Dermatologic Surgery 21(8): 669-683, 1995.
Ratner D, Nelson BR, Brown MD, et al.: Merkel cell carcinoma. Journal of the American Academy of Dermatology 29(2 part 1): 143-156, 1993.
Gould VE, Moll R, Moll I, et al.: Neuroendocrine (Merkel) cells of the skin: hyperplasias, dysplasias, and neoplasms. Laboratory Investigation 52(4): 334-353, 1985.
[40] Haag ML, Glass LF, Fenske NA: Merkel cell carcinoma. Diagnosis and treatment. Dermatologic Surgery 21(8): 669-683, 1995.

- Stage III: Presence of systemic metastases beyond the regional lymph nodes.

Treatment Option Overview

The designations in PDQ that treatments are "standard" or "under clinical evaluation" are not to be used as a basis for reimbursement determinations.

Stage I Merkel Cell Carcinoma

Wide local excision has been recommended whenever possible.[41] [Level of evidence: 3iiiD] Frozen section control has also been recommended, especially when the tumor is in an anatomical site that is not amenable to wide margins. Some authors have advocated the use of Mohs micrographic surgery as a tissue-sparing technique, but comparatively few cases have been treated in this manner.[42] The role of elective lymph node dissection (ELND) in the absence of clinically positive nodes is controversial. ELND has been recommended for larger tumors, tumors with greater than 10 mitoses per high-power field, lymphatic or vascular invasion, and the small-cell histologic subtypes.[43] There are no data available with regard to the role of sentinel lymph node mapping and biopsy in the management of MCC.

Radiation therapy to the primary site after excision and to the regional lymph node basin has been advocated by some authors;[44] however, others

---

[41] Haag ML, Glass LF, Fenske NA: Merkel cell carcinoma. Diagnosis and treatment. Dermatologic Surgery 21(8): 669-683, 1995.
Ratner D, Nelson BR, Brown MD, et al.: Merkel cell carcinoma. Journal of the American Academy of Dermatology 29(2 part 1): 143-156, 1993.
Yiengpruksawan A, Coit DG, Thaler HT, et al.: Merkel cell carcinoma. Prognosis and management. Archives of Surgery 126(12): 1514-1519, 1991.
[42] Ratner D, Nelson BR, Brown MD, et al.: Merkel cell carcinoma. Journal of the American Academy of Dermatology 29(2 part 1): 143-156, 1993.
Goepfert H, Remmler D, Silva E, et al.: Merkel cell carcinoma (endocrine carcinoma of the skin) of the head and neck. Archives of Otolaryngology, Head and Neck Surgery 110(11): 707-712, 1984.
[43] Haag ML, Glass LF, Fenske NA: Merkel cell carcinoma. Diagnosis and treatment. Dermatologic Surgery 21(8): 669-683, 1995.
Ratner D, Nelson BR, Brown MD, et al.: Merkel cell carcinoma. Journal of the American Academy of Dermatology 29(2 part 1): 143-156, 1993.
Yiengpruksawan A, Coit DG, Thaler HT, et al.: Merkel cell carcinoma. Prognosis and management. Archives of Surgery 126(12): 1514-1519, 1991.
[44] Haag ML, Glass LF, Fenske NA: Merkel cell carcinoma. Diagnosis and treatment. Dermatologic Surgery 21(8): 669-683, 1995.

have found no advantage in local or regional control with adjuvant radiation therapy in comparison with aggressive surgical therapy.[45] In general, radiation therapy has been recommended for larger tumors, those with lymphatic invasion, tumors approaching the surgical margins of resection, and locally unresectable tumors. Total doses of 40 Gy to 60 Gy to the surgical bed and the draining regional lymphatics have been used.[46] For unresected tumors or tumors with microscopic evidence of spread beyond resected margins, doses of 56 Gy to 65 Gy have been recommended.[47] [Level of evidence: 3iiiD]

Stage II Merkel Cell Carcinoma

Wide local excision of the primary tumor, whenever possible, and regional lymph node dissection have been recommended.[48] [Level of evidence: 3iiiD] Although most authors advocate the use of adjuvant radiation therapy,[49]

Ratner D, Nelson BR, Brown MD, et al.: Merkel cell carcinoma. Journal of the American Academy of Dermatology 29(2 part 1): 143-156, 1993.
Goepfert H, Remmler D, Silva E, et al.: Merkel cell carcinoma (endocrine carcinoma of the skin) of the head and neck. Archives of Otolaryngology, Head and Neck Surgery 110(11): 707-712, 1984.
Gollard R, Weber R, Kosty MP, et al.: Merkel cell carcinoma. Review of 22 cases with surgical, pathologic, and therapeutic considerations. Cancer 88(8): 1842-1851, 2000.
[45] Yiengpruksawan A, Coit DG, Thaler HT, et al.: Merkel cell carcinoma. Prognosis and management. Archives of Surgery 126(12): 1514-1519, 1991.
[46] Haag ML, Glass LF, Fenske NA: Merkel cell carcinoma. Diagnosis and treatment. Dermatologic Surgery 21(8): 669-683, 1995.
Ratner D, Nelson BR, Brown MD, et al.: Merkel cell carcinoma. Journal of the American Academy of Dermatology 29(2 part 1): 143-156, 1993.
Gollard R, Weber R, Kosty MP, et al.: Merkel cell carcinoma. Review of 22 cases with surgical, pathologic, and therapeutic considerations. Cancer 88(8): 1842-1851, 2000.
Marks ME, Kim RY, Salter MM: Radiotherapy as an adjunct in the management of Merkel cell carcinoma. Cancer 65(1): 60-64, 1990.
[47] Haag ML, Glass LF, Fenske NA: Merkel cell carcinoma. Diagnosis and treatment. Dermatologic Surgery 21(8): 669-683, 1995.
[48] Haag ML, Glass LF, Fenske NA: Merkel cell carcinoma. Diagnosis and treatment. Dermatologic Surgery 21(8): 669-683, 1995.
Yiengpruksawan A, Coit DG, Thaler HT, et al.: Merkel cell carcinoma. Prognosis and management. Archives of Surgery 126(12): 1514-1519, 1991.
[49] Haag ML, Glass LF, Fenske NA: Merkel cell carcinoma. Diagnosis and treatment. Dermatologic Surgery 21(8): 669-683, 1995.
Ratner D, Nelson BR, Brown MD, et al.: Merkel cell carcinoma. Journal of the American Academy of Dermatology 29(2 part 1): 143-156, 1993.
Goepfert H, Remmler D, Silva E, et al.: Merkel cell carcinoma (endocrine carcinoma of the skin) of the head and neck. Archives of Otolaryngology, Head and Neck Surgery 110(11): 707-712, 1984.
Marks ME, Kim RY, Salter MM: Radiotherapy as an adjunct in the management of Merkel cell carcinoma. Cancer 65(1): 60-64, 1990.

others have found no advantage in local or regional control with adjuvant radiation compared with aggressive surgery alone.[50] In general, the primary site and regional lymph node-bearing areas are included in the radiation field. The role of adjuvant chemotherapy remains unproven, but is advocated by some authors.[51] The chemotherapy regimens that have been employed are similar to those used for patients with small cell lung cancer.

Stage III Merkel Cell Carcinoma

Chemotherapy is the treatment most often used for patients with stage III Merkel cell carcinoma (MCC).[52] [Level of evidence: 3iiiDiii] Because of morphologic and immunohistochemical similarities, the regimens employed are similar to those used for patients with small cell lung cancer. MCC often responds to chemotherapy initially, but the response is usually short-lived and the impact of chemotherapy on survival is uncertain.[53]

---

[50] Yiengpruksawan A, Coit DG, Thaler HT, et al.: Merkel cell carcinoma. Prognosis and management. Archives of Surgery 126(12): 1514-1519, 1991.

[51] Haag ML, Glass LF, Fenske NA: Merkel cell carcinoma. Diagnosis and treatment. Dermatologic Surgery 21(8): 669-683, 1995.
Tai PT, Yu E, Winquist E, et al.: Chemotherapy in neuroendocrine/Merkel cell carcinoma of the skin: case series and review of 204 cases. Journal of Clinical Oncology 18(12): 2493-2499, 2000.
Feun LG, Savaraj N, Legha SS, et al.: Chemotherapy for metastatic Merkel cell carcinoma. Review of the M.D. Anderson Hospital's experience. Cancer 62(4): 683-685, 1988.

[52] Haag ML, Glass LF, Fenske NA: Merkel cell carcinoma. Diagnosis and treatment. Dermatologic Surgery 21(8): 669-683, 1995.
Ratner D, Nelson BR, Brown MD, et al.: Merkel cell carcinoma. Journal of the American Academy of Dermatology 29(2 part 1): 143-156, 1993.
Tai PT, Yu E, Winquist E, et al.: Chemotherapy in neuroendocrine/Merkel cell carcinoma of the skin: case series and review of 204 cases. Journal of Clinical Oncology 18(12): 2493-2499, 2000.
Feun LG, Savaraj N, Legha SS, et al.: Chemotherapy for metastatic Merkel cell carcinoma. Review of the M.D. Anderson Hospital's experience. Cancer 62(4): 683-685, 1988.
Voog E, Biron P, Martin JP, et al.: Chemotherapy for patients with locally advanced or metastatic Merkel cell carcinoma. Cancer 85(12): 2589-2595, 1999.

[53] Haag ML, Glass LF, Fenske NA: Merkel cell carcinoma. Diagnosis and treatment. Dermatologic Surgery 21(8): 669-683, 1995.
Ratner D, Nelson BR, Brown MD, et al.: Merkel cell carcinoma. Journal of the American Academy of Dermatology 29(2 part 1): 143-156, 1993.
Tai PT, Yu E, Winquist E, et al.: Chemotherapy in neuroendocrine/Merkel cell carcinoma of the skin: case series and review of 204 cases. Journal of Clinical Oncology 18(12): 2493-2499, 2000.
Feun LG, Savaraj N, Legha SS, et al.: Chemotherapy for metastatic Merkel cell carcinoma. Review of the M.D. Anderson Hospital's experience. Cancer 62(4): 683-685, 1988.
Voog E, Biron P, Martin JP, et al.: Chemotherapy for patients with locally advanced or metastatic Merkel cell carcinoma. Cancer 85(12): 2589-2595, 1999.

Recurrent Merkel Cell Carcinoma

Treatment options for patients with local recurrence are similar to those for patients with stage II disease because the likelihood of regional lymph node metastasis is very high.[54] Regional lymph node dissection and adjuvant radiation therapy have been advised if the regional draining nodes have not been previously treated. Chemotherapy may be an option for patients with unresectable recurrent tumors or patients who have received their maximum tolerated radiation dose.[55]

NIH Databases

In addition to the various Institutes of Health that publish professional guidelines, the NIH has designed a number of databases for professionals.[56] Physician-oriented resources provide a wide variety of information related to the biomedical and health sciences, both past and present. The format of these resources varies. Searchable databases, bibliographic citations, full text articles (when available), archival collections, and images are all available. The following are referenced by the National Library of Medicine:[57]

- **Bioethics:** Access to published literature on the ethical, legal and public policy issues surrounding healthcare and biomedical research. This information is provided in conjunction with the Kennedy Institute of Ethics located at Georgetown University, Washington, D.C.:
  http://www.nlm.nih.gov/databases/databases_bioethics.html

- **HIV/AIDS Resources:** Describes various links and databases dedicated to HIV/AIDS research:
  http://www.nlm.nih.gov/pubs/factsheets/aidsinfs.html

- **NLM Online Exhibitions:** Describes "Exhibitions in the History of Medicine": **http://www.nlm.nih.gov/exhibition/exhibition.html**.
  Additional resources for historical scholarship in medicine:
  http://www.nlm.nih.gov/hmd/hmd.html

---

[54] Haag ML, Glass LF, Fenske NA: Merkel cell carcinoma. Diagnosis and treatment. Dermatologic Surgery 21(8): 669-683, 1995.
Ratner D, Nelson BR, Brown MD, et al.: Merkel cell carcinoma. Journal of the American Academy of Dermatology 29(2 part 1): 143-156, 1993.
[55] Haag ML, Glass LF, Fenske NA: Merkel cell carcinoma. Diagnosis and treatment. Dermatologic Surgery 21(8): 669-683, 1995.
[56] Remember, for the general public, the National Library of Medicine recommends the databases referenced in MEDLINE*plus* (**http://medlineplus.gov/** or **http://www.nlm.nih.gov/medlineplus/databases.html**).
[57] See **http://www.nlm.nih.gov/databases/databases.html**.

- **Biotechnology Information:** Access to public databases. The National Center for Biotechnology Information conducts research in computational biology, develops software tools for analyzing genome data, and disseminates biomedical information for the better understanding of molecular processes affecting human health and disease: **http://www.ncbi.nlm.nih.gov/**

- **Population Information:** The National Library of Medicine provides access to worldwide coverage of population, family planning, and related health issues, including family planning technology and programs, fertility, and population law and policy: **http://www.nlm.nih.gov/databases/databases_population.html**

- **Cancer Information:** Access to caner-oriented databases: **http://www.nlm.nih.gov/databases/databases_cancer.html**

- **Profiles in Science:** Offering the archival collections of prominent twentieth-century biomedical scientists to the public through modern digital technology: **http://www.profiles.nlm.nih.gov/**

- **Chemical Information:** Provides links to various chemical databases and references: **http://sis.nlm.nih.gov/Chem/ChemMain.html**

- **Clinical Alerts:** Reports the release of findings from the NIH-funded clinical trials where such release could significantly affect morbidity and mortality: **http://www.nlm.nih.gov/databases/alerts/clinical_alerts.html**

- **Space Life Sciences:** Provides links and information to space-based research (including NASA): **http://www.nlm.nih.gov/databases/databases_space.html**

- **MEDLINE:** Bibliographic database covering the fields of medicine, nursing, dentistry, veterinary medicine, the healthcare system, and the pre-clinical sciences: **http://www.nlm.nih.gov/databases/databases_medline.html**

- **Toxicology and Environmental Health Information (TOXNET):** Databases covering toxicology and environmental health: **http://sis.nlm.nih.gov/Tox/ToxMain.html**

- **Visible Human Interface:** Anatomically detailed, three-dimensional representations of normal male and female human bodies: **http://www.nlm.nih.gov/research/visible/visible_human.html**

While all of the above references may be of interest to physicians who study and treat merkel cell carcinoma, the following are particularly noteworthy.

The Combined Health Information Database

A comprehensive source of information on clinical guidelines written for professionals is the Combined Health Information Database. You will need to limit your search to "Brochure/Pamphlet," "Fact Sheet," or "Information Package" and merkel cell carcinoma using the "Detailed Search" option. Go directly to the following hyperlink: **http://chid.nih.gov/detail/detail.html**. To find associations, use the drop boxes at the bottom of the search page where "You may refine your search by." For the publication date, select "All Years," select your preferred language, and the format option "Fact Sheet." By making these selections and typing "merkel cell carcinoma" (or synonyms) into the "For these words:" box above, you will only receive results on fact sheets dealing with merkel cell carcinoma.

The NLM Gateway[58]

The NLM (National Library of Medicine) Gateway is a Web-based system that lets users search simultaneously in multiple retrieval systems at the U.S. National Library of Medicine (NLM). It allows users of NLM services to initiate searches from one Web interface, providing "one-stop searching" for many of NLM's information resources or databases.[59] One target audience for the Gateway is the Internet user who is new to NLM's online resources and does not know what information is available or how best to search for it. This audience may include physicians and other healthcare providers, researchers, librarians, students, and, increasingly, patients, their families, and the public.[60] To use the NLM Gateway, simply go to the search site at **http://gateway.nlm.nih.gov/gw/Cmd**. Type "merkel cell carcinoma" (or synonyms) into the search box and click "Search." The results will be presented in a tabular form, indicating the number of references in each database category.

---

[58] Adapted from NLM: http://gateway.nlm.nih.gov/gw/Cmd?Overview.x.

[59] The NLM Gateway is currently being developed by the Lister Hill National Center for Biomedical Communications (LHNCBC) at the National Library of Medicine (NLM) of the National Institutes of Health (NIH).

[60] Other users may find the Gateway useful for an overall search of NLM's information resources. Some searchers may locate what they need immediately, while others will utilize the Gateway as an adjunct tool to other NLM search services such as PubMed® and MEDLINEplus®. The Gateway connects users with multiple NLM retrieval systems while also providing a search interface for its own collections. These collections include various types of information that do not logically belong in PubMed, LOCATORplus, or other established NLM retrieval systems (e.g., meeting announcements and pre-1966 journal citations). The Gateway will provide access to the information found in an increasing number of NLM retrieval systems in several phases.

Results Summary

Category	Items Found
Journal Articles	351354
Books / Periodicals / Audio Visual	2588
Consumer Health	294
Meeting Abstracts	2575
Other Collections	87
Total	356898

HSTAT[61]

HSTAT is a free, Web-based resource that provides access to full-text documents used in healthcare decision-making.[62] HSTAT's audience includes healthcare providers, health service researchers, policy makers, insurance companies, consumers, and the information professionals who serve these groups. HSTAT provides access to a wide variety of publications, including clinical practice guidelines, quick-reference guides for clinicians, consumer health brochures, evidence reports and technology assessments from the Agency for Healthcare Research and Quality (AHRQ), as well as AHRQ's Put Prevention Into Practice.[63] Simply search by "merkel cell carcinoma" (or synonyms) at the following Web site: **http://text.nlm.nih.gov**.

Coffee Break: Tutorials for Biologists[64]

Some patients may wish to have access to a general healthcare site that takes a scientific view of the news and covers recent breakthroughs in biology that may one day assist physicians in developing treatments. To this end, we

---

[61] Adapted from HSTAT: **http://www.nlm.nih.gov/pubs/factsheets/hstat.html**.
[62] The HSTAT URL is **http://hstat.nlm.nih.gov/**.
[63] Other important documents in HSTAT include: the National Institutes of Health (NIH) Consensus Conference Reports and Technology Assessment Reports; the HIV/AIDS Treatment Information Service (ATIS) resource documents; the Substance Abuse and Mental Health Services Administration's Center for Substance Abuse Treatment (SAMHSA/CSAT) Treatment Improvement Protocols (TIP) and Center for Substance Abuse Prevention (SAMHSA/CSAP) Prevention Enhancement Protocols System (PEPS); the Public Health Service (PHS) Preventive Services Task Force's *Guide to Clinical Preventive Services*; the independent, nonfederal Task Force on Community Services *Guide to Community Preventive Services*; and the Health Technology Advisory Committee (HTAC) of the Minnesota Health Care Commission (MHCC) health technology evaluations.
[64] Adapted from **http://www.ncbi.nlm.nih.gov/Coffeebreak/Archive/FAQ.html**.

recommend "Coffee Break," a collection of short reports on recent biological discoveries. Each report incorporates interactive tutorials that demonstrate how bioinformatics tools are used as a part of the research process. Currently, all Coffee Breaks are written by NCBI staff.[65] Each report is about 400 words and is usually based on a discovery reported in one or more articles from recently published, peer-reviewed literature.[66] This site has new articles every few weeks, so it can be considered an online magazine of sorts, and intended for general background information. You can access the Coffee Break Web site at the following hyperlink: **http://www.ncbi.nlm.nih.gov/Coffeebreak/**.

Other Commercial Databases

In addition to resources maintained by official agencies, other databases exist that are commercial ventures addressing medical professionals. Here are a few examples that may interest you:

- **CliniWeb International:** Index and table of contents to selected clinical information on the Internet; see **http://www.ohsu.edu/cliniweb/**.

- **Image Engine:** Multimedia electronic medical record system that integrates a wide range of digitized clinical images with textual data stored in the University of Pittsburgh Medical Center's MARS electronic medical record system; see the following Web site: **http://www.cml.upmc.edu/cml/imageengine/imageEngine.html**.

- **Medical World Search:** Searches full text from thousands of selected medical sites on the Internet; see **http://www.mwsearch.com/**.

- **MedWeaver:** Prototype system that allows users to search differential diagnoses for any list of signs and symptoms, to search medical literature, and to explore relevant Web sites; see **http://www.med.virginia.edu/~wmd4n/medweaver.html**.

- **Metaphrase:** Middleware component intended for use by both caregivers and medical records personnel. It converts the informal language generally used by caregivers into terms from formal, controlled

---

[65] The figure that accompanies each article is frequently supplied by an expert external to NCBI, in which case the source of the figure is cited. The result is an interactive tutorial that tells a biological story.

[66] After a brief introduction that sets the work described into a broader context, the report focuses on how a molecular understanding can provide explanations of observed biology and lead to therapies for diseases. Each vignette is accompanied by a figure and hypertext links that lead to a series of pages that interactively show how NCBI tools and resources are used in the research process.

vocabularies; see the following Web site: http://www.lexical.com/Metaphrase.html.

The Genome Project and Merkel Cell Carcinoma

With all the discussion in the press about the Human Genome Project, it is only natural that physicians, researchers, and patients want to know about how human genes relate to merkel cell carcinoma. In the following section, we will discuss databases and references used by physicians and scientists who work in this area.

Online Mendelian Inheritance in Man (OMIM)

The Online Mendelian Inheritance in Man (OMIM) database is a catalog of human genes and genetic disorders authored and edited by Dr. Victor A. McKusick and his colleagues at Johns Hopkins and elsewhere. OMIM was developed for the World Wide Web by the National Center for Biotechnology Information (NCBI).[67] The database contains textual information, pictures, and reference information. It also contains copious links to NCBI's Entrez database of MEDLINE articles and sequence information.

To search the database, go to http://www.ncbi.nlm.nih.gov/Omim/searchomim.html. Type "merkel cell carcinoma" (or synonyms) in the search box, and click "Submit Search." If too many results appear, you can narrow the search by adding the word "clinical." Each report will have additional links to related research and databases. By following these links, especially the link titled "Database Links," you will be exposed to numerous specialized databases that are largely used by the scientific community. These databases are overly technical and seldom used by the general public, but offer an abundance of information. The following is an example of the results you can obtain from the OMIM for merkel cell carcinoma:

---

[67] Adapted from http://www.ncbi.nlm.nih.gov/. Established in 1988 as a national resource for molecular biology information, NCBI creates public databases, conducts research in computational biology, develops software tools for analyzing genome data, and disseminates biomedical information--all for the better understanding of molecular processes affecting human health and disease.

- **Carcinoid Tumors, Intestinal**
  Web site: http://www.ncbi.nlm.nih.gov/htbin-post/Omim/dispmim?114900
- **Cowden Disease**
  Web site: http://www.ncbi.nlm.nih.gov/htbin-post/Omim/dispmim?158350
- **Paragangliomas, Familial Nonchromaffin, 1; Pgl1**
  Web site: http://www.ncbi.nlm.nih.gov/htbin-post/Omim/dispmim?168000
- **Pheochromocytoma**
  Web site: http://www.ncbi.nlm.nih.gov/htbin-post/Omim/dispmim?171300
- **Succinate Dehydrogenase Complex, Subunit D, Integral Membrane Protein**
  Web site: http://www.ncbi.nlm.nih.gov/htbin-post/Omim/dispmim?602690

Genes and Disease (NCBI - Map)

The Genes and Disease database is produced by the National Center for Biotechnology Information of the National Library of Medicine at the National Institutes of Health. This Web site categorizes each disorder by the system of the body associated with it. Go to **http://www.ncbi.nlm.nih.gov/disease/**, and browse the system pages to have a full view of important conditions linked to human genes. Since this site is regularly updated, you may wish to re-visit it from time to time. The following systems and associated disorders are addressed:

- **Cancer:** Uncontrolled cell division.
  Examples: Breast And Ovarian Cancer, Burkitt lymphoma, chronic myeloid leukemia, colon cancer, lung cancer, malignant melanoma, multiple endocrine neoplasia, neurofibromatosis, p53 tumor suppressor, pancreatic cancer, prostate cancer, Ras oncogene, RB: retinoblastoma, von Hippel-Lindau syndrome.
  Web site: **http://www.ncbi.nlm.nih.gov/disease/Cancer.html**

Entrez

Entrez is a search and retrieval system that integrates several linked databases at the National Center for Biotechnology Information (NCBI).

These databases include nucleotide sequences, protein sequences, macromolecular structures, whole genomes, and MEDLINE through PubMed. Entrez provides access to the following databases:

- **PubMed:** Biomedical literature (PubMed),
  Web site: **http://www.ncbi.nlm.nih.gov/entrez/query.fcgi?db=PubMed**

- **Nucleotide Sequence Database (Genbank):**
  Web site:
  http://www.ncbi.nlm.nih.gov/entrez/query.fcgi?db=Nucleotide

- **Protein Sequence Database:**
  Web site: **http://www.ncbi.nlm.nih.gov/entrez/query.fcgi?db=Protein**

- **Structure:** Three-dimensional macromolecular structures,
  Web site: **http://www.ncbi.nlm.nih.gov/entrez/query.fcgi?db=Structure**

- **Genome:** Complete genome assemblies,
  Web site: **http://www.ncbi.nlm.nih.gov/entrez/query.fcgi?db=Genome**

- **PopSet:** Population study data sets,
  Web site: **http://www.ncbi.nlm.nih.gov/entrez/query.fcgi?db=Popset**

- **OMIM:** Online Mendelian Inheritance in Man,
  Web site: **http://www.ncbi.nlm.nih.gov/entrez/query.fcgi?db=OMIM**

- **Taxonomy:** Organisms in GenBank,
  Web site:
  http://www.ncbi.nlm.nih.gov/entrez/query.fcgi?db=Taxonomy

- **Books:** Online books,
  Web site: **http://www.ncbi.nlm.nih.gov/entrez/query.fcgi?db=books**

- **ProbeSet:** Gene Expression Omnibus (GEO),
  Web site: **http://www.ncbi.nlm.nih.gov/entrez/query.fcgi?db=geo**

- **3D Domains:** Domains from Entrez Structure,
  Web site: **http://www.ncbi.nlm.nih.gov/entrez/query.fcgi?db=geo**

- **NCBI's Protein Sequence Information Survey Results:**
  Web site: **http://www.ncbi.nlm.nih.gov/About/proteinsurvey/**

To access the Entrez system at the National Center for Biotechnology Information, go to **http://www.ncbi.nlm.nih.gov/entrez/**, and then select the database that you would like to search. The databases available are listed in the drop box next to "Search." In the box next to "for," enter "merkel cell carcinoma" (or synonyms) and click "Go."

Jablonski's Multiple Congenital Anomaly/Mental Retardation (MCA/MR) Syndromes Database[68]

This online resource can be quite useful. It has been developed to facilitate the identification and differentiation of syndromic entities. Special attention is given to the type of information that is usually limited or completely omitted in existing reference sources due to space limitations of the printed form.

At the following Web site you can also search across syndromes using an index: **http://www.nlm.nih.gov/mesh/jablonski/syndrome_toc/toc_a.html**. You can search by keywords at this Web site: **http://www.nlm.nih.gov/mesh/jablonski/syndrome_db.html**.

The Genome Database[69]

Established at Johns Hopkins University in Baltimore, Maryland in 1990, the Genome Database (GDB) is the official central repository for genomic mapping data resulting from the Human Genome Initiative. In the spring of 1999, the Bioinformatics Supercomputing Centre (BiSC) at the Hospital for Sick Children in Toronto, Ontario assumed the management of GDB. The Human Genome Initiative is a worldwide research effort focusing on structural analysis of human DNA to determine the location and sequence of the estimated 100,000 human genes. In support of this project, GDB stores and curates data generated by researchers worldwide who are engaged in the mapping effort of the Human Genome Project (HGP). GDB's mission is to provide scientists with an encyclopedia of the human genome which is continually revised and updated to reflect the current state of scientific knowledge. Although GDB has historically focused on gene mapping, its focus will broaden as the Genome Project moves from mapping to sequence, and finally, to functional analysis.

To access the GDB, simply go to the following hyperlink: **http://www.gdb.org/**. Search "All Biological Data" by "Keyword." Type "merkel cell carcinoma" (or synonyms) into the search box, and review the results. If more than one word is used in the search box, then separate each one with the word "and" or "or" (using "or" might be useful when using synonyms). This database is extremely technical as it was created for

---

[68] Adapted from the National Library of Medicine: **http://www.nlm.nih.gov/mesh/jablonski/about_syndrome.html**.
[69] Adapted from the Genome Database:
http://gdbwww.gdb.org/gdb/aboutGDB.html#mission.

specialists. The articles are the results which are the most accessible to non-professionals and often listed under the heading "Citations." The contact names are also accessible to non-professionals.

Specialized References

The following books are specialized references written for professionals interested in merkel cell carcinoma (sorted alphabetically by title, hyperlinks provide rankings, information, and reviews at Amazon.com):

- **Advanced and Critical Care Oncology Nursing: Managing Primary Complications** by Cynthia C. Chernecky (Editor), et al; Paperback - 736 pages (September 18, 1997), W B Saunders Co; ISBN: 0721668607; http://www.amazon.com/exec/obidos/ASIN/0721668607/icongroupinterna

- **Cancer: Etiology, Diagnosis, and Treatment** by Walter J. Burdette; Paperback - 287 pages, 1st edition (January 15, 1998), McGraw Hill Text; ISBN: 0070089922; http://www.amazon.com/exec/obidos/ASIN/0070089922/icongroupinterna

- **Cancer Management: A Multidisciplinary Approach: Medical, Surgical & Radiation** by Richard Pazdur (Editor), et al; Paperback - 982 pages, 5th edition (June 15, 2001), Publisher Research & Representation, Inc.; ISBN: 1891483080; http://www.amazon.com/exec/obidos/ASIN/1891483080/icongroupinterna

- **Familial Cancer and Prevention: Molecular Epidemiology: A New Strategy Toward Cancer Control** by Joji Utsunomiya (Editor), et al; Hardcover (April 1999), Wiley-Liss; ISBN: 0471249378; http://www.amazon.com/exec/obidos/ASIN/0471249378/icongroupinterna

- **Fundamentals of Cancer Epidemiology** by Philip C. Nasca, Ph.D. (Editor), Pastides Harris, Ph.D., MPH (Editor); Hardcover - 368 pages, 1st edition (February 15, 2001), Aspen Publishers, Inc.; ISBN: 0834217767; http://www.amazon.com/exec/obidos/ASIN/0834217767/icongroupinterna

- **Helping Cancer Patients Cope: A Problem-Solving Approach** by Arthur M. Nezu (Editor), et al; Hardcover - 314 pages (December 15, 1998), American Psychological Association (APA); ISBN: 1557985332; http://www.amazon.com/exec/obidos/ASIN/1557985332/icongroupinterna

- **Quantitative Estimation and Prediction of Human Cancer Risks (Iarc Scientific Publications, 131)** by Suresh H. Moolgavkar (Editor), et al; Paperback (September 1999), Oxford University Press; ISBN: 9283221311; http://www.amazon.com/exec/obidos/ASIN/9283221311/icongroupinterna

- **Textbook of Cancer Epidemiology** by ADAMI, et al; Hardcover - 385 pages, 1st edition (July 15, 2002), Oxford University Press; ISBN: 0195109694;
  http://www.amazon.com/exec/obidos/ASIN/0195109694/icongroupinterna

Vocabulary Builder

Anatomical: Pertaining to anatomy, or to the structure of the organism. [EU]

Axons: Nerve fibers that are capable of rapidly conducting impulses away from the neuron cell body. [NIH]

Cytoplasm: The protoplasm of a cell exclusive of that of the nucleus; it consists of a continuous aqueous solution (cytosol) and the organelles and inclusions suspended in it (phaneroplasm), and is the site of most of the chemical activities of the cell. [EU]

Elective: Subject to the choice or decision of the patient or physician; applied to procedures that are advantageous to the patient but not urgent. [EU]

Necrosis: Refers to the death of living tissues. [NIH]

Recurrence: The return of cancer, at the same site as the original (primary) tumor or in another location, after the tumor had disappeared. [NIH]

Regimen: A treatment plan that specifies the dosage, the schedule, and the duration of treatment. [NIH]

Subcutaneous: Beneath the skin. [NIH]

Unresectable: Unable to be surgically removed. [NIH]

Vesicular: 1. composed of or relating to small, saclike bodies. 2. pertaining to or made up of vesicles on the skin. [EU]

PART III. APPENDICES

ABOUT PART III

Part III is a collection of appendices on general medical topics which may be of interest to patients with merkel cell carcinoma and related conditions.

APPENDIX A. RESEARCHING YOUR MEDICATIONS

Overview

There are a number of sources available on new or existing medications which could be prescribed to patients with merkel cell carcinoma. While a number of hard copy or CD-Rom resources are available to patients and physicians for research purposes, a more flexible method is to use Internet-based databases. In this chapter, we will begin with a general overview of medications. We will then proceed to outline official recommendations on how you should view your medications. You may also want to research medications that you are currently taking for other conditions as they may interact with medications for merkel cell carcinoma. Research can give you information on the side effects, interactions, and limitations of prescription drugs used in the treatment of merkel cell carcinoma. Broadly speaking, there are two sources of information on approved medications: public sources and private sources. We will emphasize free-to-use public sources.

Your Medications: The Basics[70]

The Agency for Health Care Research and Quality has published extremely useful guidelines on how you can best participate in the medication aspects of merkel cell carcinoma. Taking medicines is not always as simple as swallowing a pill. It can involve many steps and decisions each day. The AHCRQ recommends that patients with merkel cell carcinoma take part in treatment decisions. Do not be afraid to ask questions and talk about your concerns. By taking a moment to ask questions early, you may avoid problems later. Here are some points to cover each time a new medicine is prescribed:

- Ask about all parts of your treatment, including diet changes, exercise, and medicines.
- Ask about the risks and benefits of each medicine or other treatment you might receive.
- Ask how often you or your doctor will check for side effects from a given medication.

Do not hesitate to ask what is important to you about your medicines. You may want a medicine with the fewest side effects, or the fewest doses to take each day. You may care most about cost, or how the medicine might affect how you live or work. Or, you may want the medicine your doctor believes will work the best. Telling your doctor will help him or her select the best treatment for you.

Do not be afraid to "bother" your doctor with your concerns and questions about medications for merkel cell carcinoma. You can also talk to a nurse or a pharmacist. They can help you better understand your treatment plan. Feel free to bring a friend or family member with you when you visit your doctor. Talking over your options with someone you trust can help you make better choices, especially if you are not feeling well. Specifically, ask your doctor the following:

- The name of the medicine and what it is supposed to do.
- How and when to take the medicine, how much to take, and for how long.
- What food, drinks, other medicines, or activities you should avoid while taking the medicine.
- What side effects the medicine may have, and what to do if they occur.

---

[70] This section is adapted from AHCRQ: **http://www.ahcpr.gov/consumer/ncpiebro.htm**.

- If you can get a refill, and how often.
- About any terms or directions you do not understand.
- What to do if you miss a dose.
- If there is written information you can take home (most pharmacies have information sheets on your prescription medicines; some even offer large-print or Spanish versions).

Do not forget to tell your doctor about all the medicines you are currently taking (not just those for merkel cell carcinoma). This includes prescription medicines and the medicines that you buy over the counter. Then your doctor can avoid giving you a new medicine that may not work well with the medications you take now. When talking to your doctor, you may wish to prepare a list of medicines you currently take, the reason you take them, and how you take them. Be sure to include the following information for each:

- Name of medicine
- Reason taken
- Dosage
- Time(s) of day

Also include any over-the-counter medicines, such as:
- Laxatives
- Diet pills
- Vitamins
- Cold medicine
- Aspirin or other pain, headache, or fever medicine
- Cough medicine
- Allergy relief medicine
- Antacids
- Sleeping pills
- Others (include names)

Learning More about Your Medications

Because of historical investments by various organizations and the emergence of the Internet, it has become rather simple to learn about the medications your doctor has recommended for merkel cell carcinoma. One such source is the United States Pharmacopeia. In 1820, eleven physicians met in Washington, D.C. to establish the first compendium of standard drugs for the United States. They called this compendium the "U.S. Pharmacopeia (USP)." Today, the USP is a non-profit organization consisting of 800 volunteer scientists, eleven elected officials, and 400 representatives of state associations and colleges of medicine and pharmacy. The USP is located in Rockville, Maryland, and its home page is located at **www.usp.org**. The USP currently provides standards for over 3,700 medications. The resulting USP DI® Advice for the Patient® can be accessed through the National Library of Medicine of the National Institutes of Health. The database is partially derived from lists of federally approved medications in the Food and Drug Administration's (FDA) Drug Approvals database.[71]

While the FDA database is rather large and difficult to navigate, the Phamacopeia is both user-friendly and free to use. It covers more than 9,000 prescription and over-the-counter medications. To access this database, simply type the following hyperlink into your Web browser: **http://www.nlm.nih.gov/medlineplus/druginformation.html**. To view examples of a given medication (brand names, category, description, preparation, proper use, precautions, side effects, etc.), simply follow the hyperlinks indicated within the United States Pharmacopoeia (USP). It is important to read the disclaimer by the USP (**http://www.nlm.nih.gov/medlineplus/drugdisclaimer.html**) before using the information provided.

Commercial Databases

In addition to the medications listed in the USP above, a number of commercial sites are available by subscription to physicians and their institutions. You may be able to access these sources from your local medical library or your doctor's office.

---

[71] Though cumbersome, the FDA database can be freely browsed at the following site: **www.fda.gov/cder/da/da.htm**.

Reuters Health Drug Database

The Reuters Health Drug Database can be searched by keyword at the hyperlink: **http://www.reutershealth.com/frame2/drug.html**.

Mosby's GenRx

Mosby's GenRx database (also available on CD-Rom and book format) covers 45,000 drug products including generics and international brands. It provides prescribing information, drug interactions, and patient information. Information can be obtained at the following hyperlink: **http://www.genrx.com/Mosby/PhyGenRx/group.html**.

Physicians Desk Reference

The Physicians Desk Reference database (also available in CD-Rom and book format) is a full-text drug database. The database is searchable by brand name, generic name or by indication. It features multiple drug interactions reports. Information can be obtained at the following hyperlink: **http://physician.pdr.net/physician/templates/en/acl/psuser_t.htm**.

Other Web Sites

A number of additional Web sites discuss drug information. As an example, you may like to look at **www.drugs.com** which reproduces the information in the Pharmacopeia as well as commercial information. You may also want to consider the Web site of the Medical Letter, Inc. which allows users to download articles on various drugs and therapeutics for a nominal fee: **http://www.medletter.com/**.

Drug Development and Approval

The following Web sites can be valuable resources when conducting research on the development and approval of new cancer drugs:

- FDA Home Page: Search for drugs currently in development or those which have been recently approved by the FDA.
  http://redir.nci.nih.gov/cgi-bin/redir.pl?section=Cancerinfo&destURI=http://www.fda.gov/

- Cancer Liaison Program: Answers questions from the public about drug approval processes, cancer clinical trials, and access to investigational therapies.
  http://redir.nci.nih.gov/cgi-bin/redir.pl?section=Cancerinfo&destURI=http://www.fda.gov/oashi/cancer/cancer.html

- Center for Drug Evaluation and Research
  http://redir.nci.nih.gov/cgi-bin/redir.pl?section=Cancerinfo&destURI=http://www.fda.gov/cder/

- Drug Approvals by Cancer Indications (Alphabetical List)
  http://redir.nci.nih.gov/cgi-bin/redir.pl?section=Cancerinfo&destURI=http://www.fda.gov/oashi/cancer/cdrugalpha.html

- Drug Approvals by Cancer Indications (Cancer Type)
  http://redir.nci.nih.gov/cgi-bin/redir.pl?section=Cancerinfo&destURI=http://www.fda.gov/oashi/cancer/cdrugind.html

- Electronic Orange Book of Approved Drug Products
  http://redir.nci.nih.gov/cgi-bin/redir.pl?section=Cancerinfo&destURI=http://www.fda.gov/cder/ob/default.htm

- Guidance Documents for Industry: Contains an archive of documents describing FDA policies on specific topics.
  http://redir.nci.nih.gov/cgi-bin/redir.pl?section=Cancerinfo&destURI=http://www.fda.gov/cder/guidance/index.htm

- Industry Collaboration: Provides information to industry on the process for getting new drugs into clinical trials.
  http://ctep.cancer.gov/industry/index.html

- Investigator's Handbook: Provides information to investigators on specific procedures related to clinical trial development.
  http://ctep.cancer.gov/handbook/index.html

- Questions and Answers About NCI's Natural Products Branch: A fact sheet that describes the functions of this branch, which collects and analyzes specimens of plant, marine, and microbial origin for possible anticancer properties.
  http://cis.nci.nih.gov/fact/7_33.htm

Understanding the Approval Process for New Cancer Drugs[72]

Since June 1996, about 80 new cancer-related drugs, or new uses for drugs already on the market, have been approved by the U.S. Food and Drug Administration (FDA), the division of the U.S. Department of Health and Human Services charged with ensuring the safety and effectiveness of new drugs before they can go on the market. (The FDA maintains an annotated online list of drugs approved for use with cancer since 1996.) Some of these drugs treat cancer, some alleviate pain and other symptoms, and, in one case, reduce the risk of invasive cancer in people who are considered high-risk. The FDA relied on the results of clinical trials in making every one of these approvals. Without reliable information about a drug's effects on humans, it would be impossible to approve any drug for widespread use.

When considering a new drug, the FDA faces two challenges:

- First, making sure that the drug is safe and effective before it is made widely available;
- Second, ensuring that drugs which show promise are made available as quickly as possible to the people they can help.

To deal with these challenges, the FDA maintains a rigorous review process but also has measures in place to make some drugs available in special cases. This aim of this section is to acquaint you with the drug approval process and point you to other resources for learning more about it.

The Role of the Federal Drug Administration (FDA)

Approval is only one step in the drug development process. In fact, the FDA estimates that, on average, it takes eight and a half years to study and test a new drug before it can be approved for the general public. That includes early laboratory and animal testing, as well as the clinical trials that evaluate the drugs in humans. The FDA plays a key role at three main points in this process:

- Determining whether or not a new drug shows enough promise to be given to people in clinical trials

---

[72] Adapted from the NCI:
http://www.cancer.gov/clinical_trials/doc_header.aspx?viewid=d94cbfac-e478-4704-9052-d8e8a3372b56.

- Once clinical trials begin, deciding whether or not they should continue, based on reports of efficacy and adverse reactions
- When clinical trials are completed, deciding whether or not the drug can be sold to the public and what its label should say about directions for use, side effects, warnings, and the like.

To make these decisions, the FDA must review studies submitted by the drug's sponsor (usually the manufacturer), evaluate any adverse reports from preclinical studies and clinical trials (that is, reports of side effects or complications), and review the adequacy of the chemistry and manufacturing. This process is lengthy, but it is meant to ensure that only beneficial drugs with acceptable side effects will make their way into the hands of the public. At the same time, recent legislative mandates and streamlined procedures within the FDA have accelerated the approval of effective drugs, especially for serious illnesses such as cancer. In addition, specific provisions make some drugs available to patients with special needs even before the approval process is complete.

From Lab to Patient Care

By law, the Food and Drug Administration (FDA) must review all test results for new drugs to ensure that products are safe and effective for specific uses. "Safe" does not mean that the drug is free of possible adverse side effects; rather, it means that the potential benefits have been determined to outweigh any risks. The testing process begins long before the first person takes the drug, with preliminary research and animal testing.

If a drug proves promising in the lab, the drug company or sponsor must apply for FDA approval to test it in clinical trials involving people. For drugs, the application, called an Investigational New Drug (IND) Application, is sent through the Center for Drug Evaluation and Research's (CDER) IND Review Process; for biological agents, the IND is sent to the Center for Biologics Evaluation and Research (CBER). Once the IND is approved by CDER or CBER, clinical trials can begin.

If the drug makes it through the clinical trials process—that is, the studies show that it is superior to current drugs—the manufacturer must submit a New Drug Application (NDA) or (for biological agents) a Biologics License Application (BLA) to the FDA. (Biological agents, such as serums, vaccines, and cloned proteins, are manufactured from substances taken from living humans or animals.) This application must include:

- The exact chemical makeup of the drug or biologic and the mechanisms by which it is effective
- Results of animal studies
- Results of clinical trials
- How the drug or biologic is manufactured, processed, and packaged
- Quality control standards
- Samples of the product in the form(s) in which it is to be administered.

Once the FDA receives the NDA or BLA from the manufacturer or developer, the formal New Drug Application Review Process or Biologics/Product License Application Review Process begins.

For an overview of the entire process from start to finish, see the CDER's visual representation of The New Drug Development Process: Steps from Test Tube to New Drug Application Review, which is available for public viewing at the following Web address: http://www.fda.gov/cder/handbook/develop.htm.

Speed versus Safety in the Approval Process

The FDA's current goal is that no more than ten months will pass between the time that a complete application is submitted and the FDA takes action on it. But the process is not always smooth. Sometimes FDA's external advisory panels call for additional research or data. In other cases, the FDA staff asks for more information or revised studies. Some new drug approvals have taken as little as 42 days; other more difficult NDAs have spent years in the approval process.

Setting Priorities

The order in which NDAs are assessed by the FDA is determined by a classification system designed to give priority to drugs with the greatest potential benefits. All drugs that offer significant medical advances over existing therapies for any disease are considered "priority" drugs in the approval process. NDAs for cancer treatment drugs are reviewed for this status primarily by the Division of Oncology Drug Products in the FDA's Center for Drug Evaluation and Research (CDER). For Biologic License Applications (vaccines, blood products, and medicines made from animal products), the Center for Biologics Evaluation and Research (CBER) provides additional regulation and oversight.

Expert Advice

The FDA relies on a system of independent advisory committees, made up of professionals from outside the agency, for expert advice and guidance in making sound decisions about drug approval. Each committee meets as needed to weigh available evidence and assess the safety, effectiveness, and appropriate use of products considered for approval. In addition, these committees provide advice about general criteria for evaluation and scientific issues not related to specific products. The Oncologic Drugs Advisory Committee (ODAC) meets regularly to provide expert advice on cancer-related treatments and preventive drugs.

Each committee is composed of representatives from the research science and medical fields. At least one member on every advisory committee must represent the consumer perspective.

Final Approval

As the FDA looks at all the data submitted and the results of its own review, it applies two benchmark questions to each application for drug approval:

- Do the results of well-controlled studies provide substantial evidence of effectiveness?
- Do the results show the product is safe under the conditions of use in the proposed labeling? In this context, "safe" means that potential benefits have been determined to outweigh any risks.

Continued Vigilance

The FDA's responsibility for new drug treatments does not stop with final approval. The Office of Compliance in the Center for Drug Evaluation and Research (CDER) implements and tracks programs to make sure manufacturers comply with current standards and practice regulations. CDER's Office of Drug Marketing, Advertising, and Communication monitors new drug advertising to make sure it is truthful and complete. At the Center for Biologic Evaluation and Research, biologics are followed with the same vigilance after approval. And through a system called MedWatch, the FDA gets feedback from health professionals and consumers on how the new drugs are working, any adverse reactions, and potential problems in labeling and dosage.

Online FDA Resources

The following information from the FDA should help you better understand the drug approval process:

- Center for Drug Evaluation and Research: **http://www.fda.gov/cder/handbook**
- From Test Tube to Patient: New Drug Development in the U.S. – a special January 1995 issue of the magazine FDA Consumer: **http://www.fda.gov/fdac/special/newdrug/ndd_toc.html**
- Milestones in U.S. Food and Drug Law History: **http://www.fda.gov/opacom/backgrounders/miles.html**
- Drug Approvals for Cancer Indications: **http://www.fda.gov/oashi/cancer/cdrug.html**

Getting Drugs to Patients Who Need Them

Clinical trials provide the most important information used by the FDA in determining whether a new drug shows "substantial evidence of effectiveness," or whether an already-approved drug can be used effectively in new ways (for example, to treat or prevent other types of cancer, or at a different dosage). The FDA must certify that a drug has shown promise in laboratory and animal trials before human testing can begin. The trials process includes three main stages and involves continuous review, which ensures that the sponsor can stop the study early if major problems develop or unexpected levels of treatment benefit are found. As with all clinical trials, benefits and risks must be carefully weighed by the researchers conducting the study and the patients who decide to participate.

Not everyone is eligible to participate in a clinical trial. Some patients do not fit the exact requirements for studies, some have rare forms of cancer for which only a limited number of studies are underway, and others are too ill to participate. Working with the NCI and other sponsors, the FDA has established special conditions under which a patient and his or her physician can apply to receive cancer drugs that have not yet been through the approval process. In the past, these special case applications for new drugs were grouped under the name "compassionate uses." More recently, such uses have expanded to include more patients and more categories of investigational drugs.

Access to Investigational Drugs

The process of new drug development has many parts. In the United States, until a drug has been approved by the FDA, it can generally be obtained only through several mechanisms: enrollment in a clinical trial studying the drug, an expanded access program or special exemption/compassionate use programs. For more information about investigational drugs, see "Questions and Answers: Access to Investigational Drugs" at http://www.cancer.gov/cancer_information/doc_img.aspx?viewid=74b62d84-e135-451f-9bc9-d54358ede947.

"Group C" Drugs

In the 1970s, researchers from the NCI became concerned about the lag between the date when an investigational drug was found to have anti-tumor activity and the time that drug became available on the market. Working with the FDA, the NCI established the "Group C" classification to allow access to drugs with reproducible activity. Group C drugs are provided to properly trained physicians who have registered using a special form to assure that their patient qualifies under guideline protocols for the drug. Each Group C drug protocol specifies patient eligibility, reporting methodology, and drug use. Not only does Group C designation (now called Group C/Treatment INDs) speed new drugs to patients who need them most, but the process also allows the NCI to gather important information on the safety as well as activity of the drugs in the settings in which they will be most used after final FDA approval. Drugs are placed in the Group C category by agreement between the FDA and the NCI. Group C drugs are always provided free of charge, and the Health Care Financing Administration provides coverage for care associated with Group C therapy.

Treatment INDs

In 1987, the FDA began authorizing the use of new drugs still in the development process to treat certain seriously ill patients. In these cases, the process is referred to as a treatment investigational new drug application (Treatment IND). Clinical trials of the new drug must already be underway and have demonstrated positive results that are reproducible. The FDA sets guidelines about what constitutes serious and life-threatening illnesses, how much must already be known about a drug's side effects and benefits, and where physicians can obtain the drug for treatment. For many seriously ill patients, the risks associated with taking a not-yet-completely proven drug are outweighed by the possible benefits.

Accelerated Approval

"Accelerated approval" is the short-hand term for the FDA's new review system which, in the 1990s, has been used to ensure rapid approval while at the same time putting new safeguards into place. Accelerated approval is based on "surrogate endpoint" judgments: FDA can grant marketing approval to drugs and treatments that, according to certain indicators, prove they are likely to have beneficial effects on a disease or condition, even before such direct benefits have been shown clinically. Accelerated approval does NOT mean that additional clinical trials are not needed or that FDA stops gathering information about the effects of the drug; a follow-up study is required to demonstrate activity by more conventional endpoints.

Contraindications and Interactions (Hidden Dangers)

Some of the medications mentioned in the previous discussions can be problematic for patients with merkel cell carcinoma--not because they are used in the treatment process, but because of contraindications, or side effects. Medications with contraindications are those that could react with drugs used to treat merkel cell carcinoma or potentially create deleterious side effects in patients with merkel cell carcinoma. You should ask your physician about any contraindications, especially as these might apply to other medications that you may be taking for common ailments.

Drug-drug interactions occur when two or more drugs react with each other. This drug-drug interaction may cause you to experience an unexpected side effect. Drug interactions may make your medications less effective, cause unexpected side effects, or increase the action of a particular drug. Some drug interactions can even be harmful to you.

Be sure to read the label every time you use a nonprescription or prescription drug, and take the time to learn about drug interactions. These precautions may be critical to your health. You can reduce the risk of potentially harmful drug interactions and side effects with a little bit of knowledge and common sense.

Drug labels contain important information about ingredients, uses, warnings, and directions which you should take the time to read and understand. Labels also include warnings about possible drug interactions. Further, drug labels may change as new information becomes available. This is why it's especially important to read the label every time you use a medication. When your doctor prescribes a new drug, discuss all over-the-counter and prescription medications, dietary supplements, vitamins, botanicals, minerals and herbals you take as well as the foods you eat. Ask your pharmacist for the package insert for each prescription drug you take. The package insert provides more information about potential drug interactions.

A Final Warning

At some point, you may hear of alternative medications from friends, relatives, or in the news media. Advertisements may suggest that certain alternative drugs can produce positive results for patients with merkel cell carcinoma. Exercise caution--some of these drugs may have fraudulent claims, and others may actually hurt you. The Food and Drug Administration (FDA) is the official U.S. agency charged with discovering which medications are likely to improve the health of patients with merkel cell carcinoma. The FDA warns patients to watch out for[73]:

- Secret formulas (real scientists share what they know)
- Amazing breakthroughs or miracle cures (real breakthroughs don't happen very often; when they do, real scientists do not call them amazing or miracles)
- Quick, painless, or guaranteed cures
- If it sounds too good to be true, it probably isn't true.

If you have any questions about any kind of medical treatment, the FDA may have an office near you. Look for their number in the blue pages of the phone book. You can also contact the FDA through its toll-free number, 1-888-INFO-FDA (1-888-463-6332), or on the World Wide Web at **www.fda.gov**.

---

[73] This section has been adapted from **http://www.fda.gov/opacom/lowlit/medfraud.html**

General References

In addition to the resources provided earlier in this chapter, the following general references describe medications (sorted alphabetically by title; hyperlinks provide rankings, information and reviews at Amazon.com):

- **Antifolate Drugs in Cancer Therapy (Cancer Drug Discovery and Development)** by Ann L. Jackman (Editor); Hardcover: 480 pages; (March 1999), Humana Press; ISBN: 0896035964;
http://www.amazon.com/exec/obidos/ASIN/0896035964/icongroupinterna

- **Consumers Guide to Cancer Drugs** by Gail M. Wilkes, et al; Paperback - 448 pages, 1st edition (January 15, 2000), Jones & Bartlett Publishing; ISBN: 0763711705;
http://www.amazon.com/exec/obidos/ASIN/0763711705/icongroupinterna

- **Patient Education Guide to Oncology Drugs (Book with CD-ROM)** by Gail M. Wilkes, et al; CD-ROM - 447 pages, 1st edition (January 15, 2000), Jones & Bartlett Publishing; ISBN: 076371173X;
http://www.amazon.com/exec/obidos/ASIN/076371173X/icongroupinterna

- **The Role of Multiple Intensification in Medical Oncology** by M. S. Aapro (Editor), D. Maraninchi (Editor); Hardcover (June 1998), Springer Verlag; ISBN: 3540635432;
http://www.amazon.com/exec/obidos/ASIN/3540635432/icongroupinterna

Vocabulary Builder

The following vocabulary builder gives definitions of words used in this chapter that have not been defined in previous chapters:

Aspirin: A drug that reduces pain, fever, inflammation, and blood clotting. Aspirin belongs to the family of drugs called nonsteroidal anti-inflammatory agents. It is also being studied in cancer prevention. [NIH]

Serum: The clear liquid part of the blood that remains after blood cells and clotting proteins have been removed. [NIH]

Vaccine: A substance or group of substances meant to cause the immune system to respond to a tumor or to microorganisms, such as bacteria or viruses. [NIH]

APPENDIX B. RESEARCHING ALTERNATIVE MEDICINE

Overview[74]

Research indicates that the use of complementary and alternative therapies is increasing. A large-scale study published in the November 11, 1998, issue of the Journal of the American Medical Association found that CAM use among the general public increased from 34 percent in 1990 to 42 percent in 1997.

Several surveys of CAM use by cancer patients have been conducted with small numbers of patients. One study published in the February 2000 issue of the journal *Cancer* reported that 37 percent of 46 patients with prostate cancer used one or more CAM therapies as part of their cancer treatment. These therapies included herbal remedies, old-time remedies, vitamins, and special diets. A larger study of CAM use in patients with different types of cancer was published in the July 2000 issue of the Journal of Clinical Oncology . That study found that 83 percent of 453 cancer patients had used at least one CAM therapy as part of their cancer treatment. The study included CAM therapies such as special diets, psychotherapy, spiritual practices, and vitamin supplements. When psychotherapy and spiritual practices were excluded, 69 percent of patients had used at least one CAM therapy in their cancer treatment.

In this chapter, we will begin by giving you a broad perspective on complementary and alternative therapies. Next, we will introduce you to official information sources on CAM relating to merkel cell carcinoma. Finally, at the conclusion of this chapter, we will provide a list of readings on merkel cell carcinoma from various authors. We will begin, however, with

---

[74] Adapted from the NCI: **http://cis.nci.nih.gov/fact/9_14.htm**.

the National Center for Complementary and Alternative Medicine's (NCCAM) overview of complementary and alternative medicine.

What Is CAM?[75]

Complementary and alternative medicine (CAM) covers a broad range of healing philosophies, approaches, and therapies. Generally, it is defined as those treatments and healthcare practices which are not taught in medical schools, used in hospitals, or reimbursed by medical insurance companies. Many CAM therapies are termed "holistic," which generally means that the healthcare practitioner considers the whole person, including physical, mental, emotional, and spiritual health. Some of these therapies are also known as "preventive," which means that the practitioner educates and treats the person to prevent health problems from arising, rather than treating symptoms after problems have occurred.

People use CAM treatments and therapies in a variety of ways. Therapies are used alone (often referred to as alternative), in combination with other alternative therapies, or in addition to conventional treatment (sometimes referred to as complementary). Complementary and alternative medicine, or "integrative medicine," includes a broad range of healing philosophies, approaches, and therapies. Some approaches are consistent with physiological principles of Western medicine, while others constitute healing systems with non-Western origins. While some therapies are far outside the realm of accepted Western medical theory and practice, others are becoming established in mainstream medicine.

Complementary and alternative therapies are used in an effort to prevent illness, reduce stress, prevent or reduce side effects and symptoms, or control or cure disease. Some commonly used methods of complementary or alternative therapy include mind/body control interventions such as visualization and relaxation, manual healing including acupressure and massage, homeopathy, vitamins or herbal products, and acupuncture.

Should you wish to explore non-traditional types of treatment, be sure to discuss all issues concerning treatments and therapies with your healthcare provider, whether a physician or practitioner of complementary and alternative medicine. Competent healthcare management requires knowledge of both conventional and alternative therapies you are taking for the practitioner to have a complete picture of your treatment plan.

---

[75] Adapted from the NCCAM: **http://nccam.nih.gov/nccam/fcp/faq/index.html#what-is**.

The decision to use complementary and alternative treatments is an important one. Consider before selecting an alternative therapy, the safety and effectiveness of the therapy or treatment, the expertise and qualifications of the healthcare practitioner, and the quality of delivery. These topics should be considered when selecting any practitioner or therapy.

What Are the Domains of Alternative Medicine?[76]

The list of CAM practices changes continually. The reason being is that these new practices and therapies are often proved to be safe and effective, and therefore become generally accepted as "mainstream" healthcare practices. Today, CAM practices may be grouped within five major domains: (1) alternative medical systems, (2) mind-body interventions, (3) biologically-based treatments, (4) manipulative and body-based methods, and (5) energy therapies. The individual systems and treatments comprising these categories are too numerous to list in this sourcebook. Thus, only limited examples are provided within each.

Alternative Medical Systems

Alternative medical systems involve complete systems of theory and practice that have evolved independent of, and often prior to, conventional biomedical approaches. Many are traditional systems of medicine that are practiced by individual cultures throughout the world, including a number of venerable Asian approaches.

Traditional oriental medicine emphasizes the balance or disturbances of qi (pronounced chi) or vital energy in health and disease, respectively. Traditional oriental medicine consists of a group of techniques and methods including acupuncture, herbal medicine, oriental massage, and qi gong (a form of energy therapy). Acupuncture involves stimulating specific anatomic points in the body for therapeutic purposes, usually by puncturing the skin with a thin needle.

Ayurveda is India's traditional system of medicine. Ayurvedic medicine (meaning "science of life") is a comprehensive system of medicine that places equal emphasis on body, mind, and spirit. Ayurveda strives to restore the innate harmony of the individual. Some of the primary Ayurvedic

---

[76] Adapted from the NCCAM: **http://nccam.nih.gov/nccam/fcp/classify/index.html**

treatments include diet, exercise, meditation, herbs, massage, exposure to sunlight, and controlled breathing.

Other traditional healing systems have been developed by the world's indigenous populations. These populations include Native American, Aboriginal, African, Middle Eastern, Tibetan, and Central and South American cultures. Homeopathy and naturopathy are also examples of complete alternative medicine systems.

Homeopathic medicine is an unconventional Western system that is based on the principle that "like cures like," i.e., that the same substance that in large doses produces the symptoms of an illness, in very minute doses cures it. Homeopathic health practitioners believe that the more dilute the remedy, the greater its potency. Therefore, they use small doses of specially prepared plant extracts and minerals to stimulate the body's defense mechanisms and healing processes in order to treat illness.

Naturopathic medicine is based on the theory that disease is a manifestation of alterations in the processes by which the body naturally heals itself and emphasizes health restoration rather than disease treatment. Naturopathic physicians employ an array of healing practices, including the following: diet and clinical nutrition, homeopathy, acupuncture, herbal medicine, hydrotherapy (the use of water in a range of temperatures and methods of applications), spinal and soft-tissue manipulation, physical therapies (such as those involving electrical currents, ultrasound, and light), therapeutic counseling, and pharmacology.

Mind-Body Interventions

Mind-body interventions employ a variety of techniques designed to facilitate the mind's capacity to affect bodily function and symptoms. Only a select group of mind-body interventions having well-documented theoretical foundations are considered CAM. For example, patient education and cognitive-behavioral approaches are now considered "mainstream." On the other hand, complementary and alternative medicine includes meditation, certain uses of hypnosis, dance, music, and art therapy, as well as prayer and mental healing.

Biological-Based Therapies

This category of CAM includes natural and biological-based practices, interventions, and products, many of which overlap with conventional medicine's use of dietary supplements. This category includes herbal, special dietary, orthomolecular, and individual biological therapies.

Herbal therapy employs an individual herb or a mixture of herbs for healing purposes. An herb is a plant or plant part that produces and contains chemical substances that act upon the body. Special diet therapies, such as those proposed by Drs. Atkins, Ornish, Pritikin, and Weil, are believed to prevent and/or control illness as well as promote health. Orthomolecular therapies aim to treat disease with varying concentrations of chemicals such as magnesium, melatonin, and mega-doses of vitamins. Biological therapies include, for example, the use of laetrile and shark cartilage to treat cancer and the use of bee pollen to treat autoimmune and inflammatory diseases.

Manipulative and Body-Based Methods

This category includes methods that are based on manipulation and/or movement of the body. For example, chiropractors focus on the relationship between structure and function, primarily pertaining to the spine, and how that relationship affects the preservation and restoration of health. Chiropractors use manipulative therapy as an integral treatment tool.

In contrast, osteopaths place particular emphasis on the musculoskeletal system and practice osteopathic manipulation. Osteopaths believe that all of the body's systems work together and that disturbances in one system may have an impact upon function elsewhere in the body. Massage therapists manipulate the soft tissues of the body to normalize those tissues.

Energy Therapies

Energy therapies focus on energy fields originating within the body (biofields) or those from other sources (electromagnetic fields). Biofield therapies are intended to affect energy fields (the existence of which is not yet experimentally proven) that surround and penetrate the human body. Some forms of energy therapy manipulate biofields by applying pressure and/or manipulating the body by placing the hands in or through these fields. Examples include Qi gong, Reiki and Therapeutic Touch.

Qi gong is a component of traditional oriental medicine that combines movement, meditation, and regulation of breathing to enhance the flow of vital energy (qi) in the body, improve blood circulation, and enhance immune function. Reiki, the Japanese word representing Universal Life Energy, is based on the belief that, by channeling spiritual energy through the practitioner, the spirit is healed and, in turn, heals the physical body. Therapeutic Touch is derived from the ancient technique of "laying-on of hands." It is based on the premises that the therapist's healing force affects the patient's recovery and that healing is promoted when the body's energies are in balance. By passing their hands over the patient, these healers identify energy imbalances.

Bioelectromagnetic-based therapies involve the unconventional use of electromagnetic fields to treat illnesses or manage pain. These therapies are often used to treat asthma, cancer, and migraine headaches. Types of electromagnetic fields which are manipulated in these therapies include pulsed fields, magnetic fields, and alternating current or direct current fields.

Research indicates that the use of complementary and alternative therapies is increasing. A large-scale study published in the November 11, 1998, issue of the Journal of the American Medical Association found that CAM use among the general public increased from 34 percent in 1990 to 42 percent in 1997.

Several surveys of CAM use by cancer patients have been conducted with small numbers of patients. One study published in the February 2000 issue of the journal Cancer reported that 37 percent of 46 patients with prostate cancer used one or more CAM therapies as part of their cancer treatment. These therapies included herbal remedies, old-time remedies, vitamins, and special diets. A larger study of CAM use in patients with different types of cancer was published in the July 2000 issue of the Journal of Clinical Oncology . That study found that 83 percent of 453 cancer patients had used at least one CAM therapy as part of their cancer treatment. The study included CAM therapies such as special diets, psychotherapy, spiritual practices, and vitamin supplements. When psychotherapy and spiritual practices were excluded, 69 percent of patients had used at least one CAM therapy in their cancer treatment.

How Are Complementary and Alternative Approaches Evaluated?[77]

It is important that the same scientific evaluation which is used to assess conventional approaches be used to evaluate complementary and alternative therapies. A number of medical centers are evaluating complementary and alternative therapies by developing clinical trials (research studies with people) to test them.

Conventional approaches to cancer treatment have generally been studied for safety and effectiveness through a rigorous scientific process, including clinical trials with large numbers of patients. Often, less is known about the safety and effectiveness of complementary and alternative methods. Some of these complementary and alternative therapies have not undergone rigorous evaluation. Others, once considered unorthodox, are finding a place in cancer treatment—not as cures, but as complementary therapies that may help patients feel better and recover faster. One example is acupuncture. According to a panel of experts at a National Institutes of Health (NIH) Consensus Conference in November 1997, acupuncture has been found to be effective in the management of chemotherapy-associated nausea and vomiting and in controlling pain associated with surgery. Some approaches, such as laetrile, have been studied and found ineffective or potentially harmful.

NCI-Sponsored Clinical Trials in Complementary and Alternative Medicine

The NCI is currently sponsoring several clinical trials (research studies with patients) that study complementary and alternative treatments for cancer. Current trials include enzyme therapy with nutritional support for the treatment of inoperable pancreatic cancer, shark cartilage therapy for the treatment of non-small cell lung cancer, and studies of the effects of diet on prostate and breast cancers. Some of these trials compare alternative therapies with conventional treatments, while others study the effects of complementary approaches used in addition to conventional treatments. Patients who are interested in taking part in these or any clinical trials should talk with their doctor.

More information about clinical trials sponsored by the NCI can be obtained from NCCAM (http://nccam.nih.gov, 1-888-644-6226), OCCAM

---

[77] Adapted from the NCI: **http://cis.nci.nih.gov/fact/9_14.htm**

(http://occam.nci.nih.gov), and the NCI's Cancer Information Service (CIS) (http://cis.nci.nih.gov, 1-800-4-CANCER).

Questions to Ask Your Healthcare Provider about CAM

When considering complementary and alternative therapies, ask your healthcare provider the following questions:

- What benefits can be expected from this therapy?
- What are the risks associated with this therapy?
- Do the known benefits outweigh the risks?
- What side effects can be expected?
- Will the therapy interfere with conventional treatment?
- Is this therapy part of a clinical trial? If so, who is sponsoring the trial?
- Will the therapy be covered by health insurance?
- How can patients and their health care providers learn more about complementary and alternative therapies?

Finding CAM References on Merkel Cell Carcinoma

Having read the previous discussion, you may be wondering which complementary or alternative treatments might be appropriate for merkel cell carcinoma. For the remainder of this chapter, we will direct you to a number of official sources which can assist you in researching studies and publications. Some of these articles are rather technical, so some patience may be required.

National Center for Complementary and Alternative Medicine

The National Center for Complementary and Alternative Medicine (NCCAM) of the National Institutes of Health (http://nccam.nih.gov) has created a link to the National Library of Medicine's databases to allow patients to search for articles that specifically relate to merkel cell carcinoma and complementary medicine. To search the database, go to the following Web site: **www.nlm.nih.gov/nccam/camonpubmed.html**. Select "CAM on PubMed." Enter "merkel cell carcinoma" (or synonyms) into the search box. Click "Go." The following references provide information on particular aspects of complementary and alternative medicine (CAM) that are related to merkel cell carcinoma:

- **Analysis of toxicity of Merkel cell carcinoma of the skin treated with synchronous carboplatin/etoposide and radiation: a Trans-Tasman Radiation Oncology Group study.**
  Author(s): Poulsen M, Rischin D, Walpole E, Harvey J, Macintosh J, Ainslie J, Hamilton C, Keller J, Tripcony L.
  Source: International Journal of Radiation Oncology, Biology, Physics. 2001 September 1; 51(1): 156-63.
  http://www.ncbi.nlm.nih.gov:80/entrez/query.fcgi?cmd=Retrieve&db=PubMed&list_uids=11516865&dopt=Abstract

- **Chemotherapy for Merkel cell carcinoma with carboplatin and etoposide.**
  Author(s): Pectasides D, Moutzourides G, Dimitriadis M, Varthalitis J, Athanassiou A.
  Source: American Journal of Clinical Oncology : the Official Publication of the American Radium Society. 1995 October; 18(5): 418-20.
  http://www.ncbi.nlm.nih.gov:80/entrez/query.fcgi?cmd=Retrieve&db=PubMed&list_uids=7572759&dopt=Abstract

- **Chemotherapy for metastatic Merkel cell carcinoma.**
  Author(s): George TK, di Sant'agnese PA, Bennett JM.
  Source: Cancer. 1985 September 1; 56(5): 1034-8.
  http://www.ncbi.nlm.nih.gov:80/entrez/query.fcgi?cmd=Retrieve&db=PubMed&list_uids=2990663&dopt=Abstract

- **Chemotherapy of disseminated Merkel-cell carcinoma.**
  Author(s): Redmond J III, Perry J, Sowray P, Vukelja SJ, Dawson N.
  Source: American Journal of Clinical Oncology : the Official Publication of the American Radium Society. 1991 August; 14(4): 305-7.
  http://www.ncbi.nlm.nih.gov:80/entrez/query.fcgi?cmd=Retrieve&db=PubMed&list_uids=1862761&dopt=Abstract

- **Chemotherapy of metastatic Merkel cell carcinoma: case report and review of the literature.**
  Author(s): Sharma D, Flora G, Grunberg SM.
  Source: American Journal of Clinical Oncology : the Official Publication of the American Radium Society. 1991 April; 14(2): 166-9. Review.
  http://www.ncbi.nlm.nih.gov:80/entrez/query.fcgi?cmd=Retrieve&db=PubMed&list_uids=2028925&dopt=Abstract

- **Diagnostic pitfalls of Merkel cell carcinoma and dramatic response to chemotherapy.**
  Author(s): Chang SF, Suh JW, Choi JH, Yoon GS, Huh J, Sung KJ, Moon KC, Kim WG, Koh JK.
  Source: J Dermatol. 1998 May; 25(5): 322-8.
  http://www.ncbi.nlm.nih.gov:80/entrez/query.fcgi?cmd=Retrieve&db=PubMed&list_uids=9640886&dopt=Abstract

- **Further insights into the natural history and management of primary cutaneous neuroendocrine (Merkel cell) carcinoma.**
  Author(s): Boyle F, Pendlebury S, Bell D.
  Source: International Journal of Radiation Oncology, Biology, Physics. 1995 January 15; 31(2): 315-23.
  http://www.ncbi.nlm.nih.gov:80/entrez/query.fcgi?cmd=Retrieve&db=PubMed&list_uids=7836085&dopt=Abstract

- **Merkel cell carcinoma of the scalp: dramatic resolution with primary chemotherapy.**
  Author(s): Ferrau F, Micali G, Guitart J.
  Source: Journal of the American Academy of Dermatology. 1994 August; 31(2 Pt 1): 271-2. No Abstract Available.
  http://www.ncbi.nlm.nih.gov:80/entrez/query.fcgi?cmd=Retrieve&db=PubMed&list_uids=8040414&dopt=Abstract

- **Oral etoposide for Merkel cell carcinoma in patients previously treated with intravenous etoposide.**
  Author(s): Fenig E, Brenner B, Njuguna E, Katz A, Schachter J, Sulkes A.
  Source: American Journal of Clinical Oncology : the Official Publication of the American Radium Society. 2000 February; 23(1): 65-7.
  http://www.ncbi.nlm.nih.gov:80/entrez/query.fcgi?cmd=Retrieve&db=PubMed&list_uids=10683081&dopt=Abstract

- **Pharmacokinetics of carboplatin and etoposide in a haemodialysis patient with Merkel-cell carcinoma.**
  Author(s): Suzuki S, Koide M, Sakamoto S, Matsuo T.
  Source: Nephrology, Dialysis, Transplantation : Official Publication of the European Dialysis and Transplant Association - European Renal Association. 1997 January; 12(1): 137-40.
  http://www.ncbi.nlm.nih.gov:80/entrez/query.fcgi?cmd=Retrieve&db=PubMed&list_uids=9027788&dopt=Abstract

- **The effect of aloe emodin on the proliferation of a new merkel carcinoma cell line.**
  Author(s): Wasserman L, Avigad S, Beery E, Nordenberg J, Fenig E.
  Source: The American Journal of Dermatopathology. 2002 February; 24(1): 17-22.
  http://www.ncbi.nlm.nih.gov:80/entrez/query.fcgi?cmd=Retrieve&db=PubMed&list_uids=11803275&dopt=Abstract

- **The role of radiation therapy and chemotherapy in the treatment of Merkel cell carcinoma.**
  Author(s): Fenig E, Brenner B, Katz A, Rakovsky E, Hana MB, Sulkes A.
  Source: Cancer. 1997 September 1; 80(5): 881-5.
  http://www.ncbi.nlm.nih.gov:80/entrez/query.fcgi?cmd=Retrieve&db=PubMed&list_uids=9307187&dopt=Abstract

- **The use of VP16 and cisplatin in the treatment of Merkel cell carcinoma.**
  Author(s): Davis MP, Miller EM, Rau RC, Johnson OE, Naille RA, Crnkovich MJ.
  Source: J Dermatol Surg Oncol. 1990 March; 16(3): 276-8.
  http://www.ncbi.nlm.nih.gov:80/entrez/query.fcgi?cmd=Retrieve&db=PubMed&list_uids=2312900&dopt=Abstract

- **Transient complete remission of metastasized Merkel cell carcinoma by high-dose polychemotherapy and autologous peripheral blood stem cell transplantation.**
  Author(s): Waldmann V, Goldschmidt H, Jackel A, Deichmann M, Hegenbart U, Hartschuh W, Ho A, Naher H.
  Source: The British Journal of Dermatology. 2000 October; 143(4): 837-9.
  http://www.ncbi.nlm.nih.gov:80/entrez/query.fcgi?cmd=Retrieve&db=PubMed&list_uids=11069467&dopt=Abstract

- **VP-16, cisplatin, doxorubicin, and bleomycin in metastatic Merkel cell carcinoma. Report of a case with long-term remission.**
  Author(s): Azagury M, Chevallier B, Atlan D, Graic Y, Dayot JP, Thomine E.
  Source: American Journal of Clinical Oncology : the Official Publication of the American Radium Society. 1993 April; 16(2): 102-4.
  http://www.ncbi.nlm.nih.gov:80/entrez/query.fcgi?cmd=Retrieve&db=PubMed&list_uids=7680840&dopt=Abstract

Additional Web Resources

A number of additional Web sites offer encyclopedic information covering CAM and related topics. The following is a representative sample:

- Alternative Medicine Foundation, Inc.: **http://www.herbmed.org/**
- AOL: **http://search.aol.com/cat.adp?id=169&layer=&from=subcats**
- Chinese Medicine: **http://www.newcenturynutrition.com/**
- drkoop.com®: **http://www.drkoop.com/InteractiveMedicine/IndexC.html**
- Family Village: **http://www.familyvillage.wisc.edu/med_altn.htm**
- Google: **http://directory.google.com/Top/Health/Alternative/**
- Healthnotes: **http://www.thedacare.org/healthnotes/**
- Open Directory Project: **http://dmoz.org/Health/Alternative/**
- TPN.com: **http://www.tnp.com/**
- Yahoo.com: **http://dir.yahoo.com/Health/Alternative_Medicine/**
- WebMD®Health: **http://my.webmd.com/drugs_and_herbs**
- WellNet: **http://www.wellnet.ca/herbsa-c.htm**
- WholeHealthMD.com: **http://www.wholehealthmd.com/reflib/0,1529,,00.html**

General References

A good place to find general background information on CAM is the National Library of Medicine. It has prepared within the MEDLINEplus system an information topic page dedicated to complementary and alternative medicine. To access this page, go to the MEDLINEplus site at: **www.nlm.nih.gov/medlineplus/alternativemedicine.html.** This Web site provides a general overview of various topics and can lead to a number of general sources. The following additional references describe, in broad terms, alternative and complementary medicine (sorted alphabetically by title; hyperlinks provide rankings, information, and reviews at Amazon.com):

- **Alternative Medicine Definitive Guide to Cancer** by W. John Diamond, et al; Hardcover - 1120 pages Package edition (March 18, 1997),

Alternativemedicine.Com Books; ISBN: 1887299017;
http://www.amazon.com/exec/obidos/ASIN/1887299017/icongroupinterna

- **Beating Cancer With Nutrition - Revised** by Patrick Quillin, Noreen Quillin (Contributor); Paperback - 352 pages; Book & CD edition (January 1, 2001), Bookworld Services; ISBN: 0963837281;
http://www.amazon.com/exec/obidos/ASIN/0963837281/icongroupinterna

- **Cancer: Increasing Your Odds for Survival - A Resource Guide for Integrating Mainstream, Alternative and Complementary Therapies** by David Bognar, Walter Cronkite; Paperback (August 1998), Hunter House; ISBN: 0897932471;
http://www.amazon.com/exec/obidos/ASIN/0897932471/icongroupinterna

- **Choices in Healing** by Michael Lerner; Paperback - 696 pages; (February 28, 1996), MIT Press; ISBN: 0262621045;
http://www.amazon.com/exec/obidos/ASIN/0262621045/icongroupinterna

- **The Gerson Therapy: The Amazing Nutritional Program for Cancer and Other Illnesses** by Charlotte Gerson, Morton Walker, D.P.M.; Paperback - 448 pages (October 2001), Kensington Publishing Corp.; ISBN: 1575666286;
http://www.amazon.com/exec/obidos/ASIN/1575666286/icongroupinterna

- **Natural Compounds in Cancer Therapy** by John C. Boik; Paperback - 520 pages (March 2001), Oregon Medical Press; ISBN: 0964828014;
http://www.amazon.com/exec/obidos/ASIN/0964828014/icongroupinterna

- **There's No Place Like Hope: A Guide to Beating Cancer in Mind-Sized Bites** by Vickie Girard, Dan Zadra (Editor); Hardcover - 161 pages (April 2001), Compendium Inc.; ISBN: 1888387416;
http://www.amazon.com/exec/obidos/ASIN/1888387416/icongroupinterna

- **Your Life in Your Hands** by Jane A. Plant, Ph.D; Hardcover - 272 pages (December 13, 2000), St. Martins Press (Trade); ISBN: 0312275617;
http://www.amazon.com/exec/obidos/ASIN/0312275617/icongroupinterna

For additional information on complementary and alternative medicine, ask your doctor or write to:

National Institutes of Health
National Center for Complementary and Alternative Medicine Clearinghouse
P. O. Box 8218
Silver Spring, MD 20907-8218

Vocabulary Builder

The following vocabulary builder gives definitions of words used in this chapter that have not been defined in previous chapters:

Bleomycin: An anticancer drug that belongs to the family of drugs called antitumor antibiotics. [NIH]

Cisplatin: An anticancer drug that belongs to the family of drugs called platinum compounds. [NIH]

Doxorubicin: An anticancer drug that belongs to the family of drugs called antitumor antibiotics. It is an anthracycline. [NIH]

Emodin: Purgative anthraquinone found in several plants, especially Rhamnus frangula. It was formerly used as a laxative, but is now used mainly as tool in toxicity studies. [NIH]

Enzyme: A protein that speeds up chemical reactions in the body. [NIH]

Haemodialysis: The removal of certain elements from the blood by virtue of the difference in the rates of their diffusion through a semipermeable membrane, e.g., by means of a haemodialyzer. [EU]

Inoperable: Not suitable to be operated upon. [EU]

Nausea: An unpleasant sensation, vaguely referred to the epigastrium and abdomen, and often culminating in vomiting. [EU]

Nephrology: A subspecialty of internal medicine concerned with the anatomy, physiology, and pathology of the kidney. [NIH]

Non-small cell lung cancer: A group of lung cancers that includes squamous cell carcinoma, adenocarcinoma, and large cell carcinoma. [NIH]

Psychotherapy: A generic term for the treatment of mental illness or emotional disturbances primarily by verbal or nonverbal communication. [NIH]

Remission: A decrease in or disappearance of signs and symptoms of cancer. In partial remission, some, but not all, signs and symptoms of cancer have disappeared. In complete remission, all signs and symptoms of cancer have disappeared, although there still may be cancer in the body. [NIH]

APPENDIX C. RESEARCHING NUTRITION

Overview

Since the time of Hippocrates, doctors have understood the importance of diet and nutrition to patients' health and well-being. Since then, they have accumulated an impressive archive of studies and knowledge dedicated to this subject. Based on their experience, doctors and healthcare providers may recommend particular dietary supplements to patients with merkel cell carcinoma. Any dietary recommendation is based on a patient's age, body mass, gender, lifestyle, eating habits, food preferences, and health condition. It is therefore likely that different patients with merkel cell carcinoma may be given different recommendations. Some recommendations may be directly related to merkel cell carcinoma, while others may be more related to the patient's general health. These recommendations, themselves, may differ from what official sources recommend for the average person.

In this chapter we will begin by briefly reviewing the essentials of diet and nutrition that will broadly frame more detailed discussions of merkel cell carcinoma. We will then show you how to find studies dedicated specifically to nutrition and merkel cell carcinoma.

Food and Nutrition: General Principles

What Are Essential Foods?

Food is generally viewed by official sources as consisting of six basic elements: (1) fluids, (2) carbohydrates, (3) protein, (4) fats, (5) vitamins, and (6) minerals. Consuming a combination of these elements is considered to be a healthy diet:

- **Fluids** are essential to human life as 80-percent of the body is composed of water. Water is lost via urination, sweating, diarrhea, vomiting, diuretics (drugs that increase urination), caffeine, and physical exertion.

- **Carbohydrates** are the main source for human energy (thermoregulation) and the bulk of typical diets. They are mostly classified as being either simple or complex. Simple carbohydrates include sugars which are often consumed in the form of cookies, candies, or cakes. Complex carbohydrates consist of starches and dietary fibers. Starches are consumed in the form of pastas, breads, potatoes, rice, and other foods. Soluble fibers can be eaten in the form of certain vegetables, fruits, oats, and legumes. Insoluble fibers include brown rice, whole grains, certain fruits, wheat bran and legumes.

- **Proteins** are eaten to build and repair human tissues. Some foods that are high in protein are also high in fat and calories. Food sources for protein include nuts, meat, fish, cheese, and other dairy products.

- **Fats** are consumed for both energy and the absorption of certain vitamins. There are many types of fats, with many general publications recommending the intake of unsaturated fats or those low in cholesterol.

Vitamins and minerals are fundamental to human health, growth, and, in some cases, disease prevention. Most are consumed in your diet (exceptions being vitamins K and D which are produced by intestinal bacteria and sunlight on the skin, respectively). Each vitamin and mineral plays a different role in health. The following outlines essential vitamins:

- **Vitamin A** is important to the health of your eyes, hair, bones, and skin; sources of vitamin A include foods such as eggs, carrots, and cantaloupe.

- **Vitamin B^1**, also known as thiamine, is important for your nervous system and energy production; food sources for thiamine include meat, peas, fortified cereals, bread, and whole grains.

- **Vitamin B^2**, also known as riboflavin, is important for your nervous system and muscles, but is also involved in the release of proteins from nutrients; food sources for riboflavin include dairy products, leafy vegetables, meat, and eggs.

- **Vitamin B^3**, also known as niacin, is important for healthy skin and helps the body use energy; food sources for niacin include peas, peanuts, fish, and whole grains
- **Vitamin B^6**, also known as pyridoxine, is important for the regulation of cells in the nervous system and is vital for blood formation; food sources for pyridoxine include bananas, whole grains, meat, and fish.
- **Vitamin B^{12}** is vital for a healthy nervous system and for the growth of red blood cells in bone marrow; food sources for vitamin B^{12} include yeast, milk, fish, eggs, and meat.
- **Vitamin C** allows the body's immune system to fight various diseases, strengthens body tissue, and improves the body's use of iron; food sources for vitamin C include a wide variety of fruits and vegetables.
- **Vitamin D** helps the body absorb calcium which strengthens bones and teeth; food sources for vitamin D include oily fish and dairy products.
- **Vitamin E** can help protect certain organs and tissues from various degenerative diseases; food sources for vitamin E include margarine, vegetables, eggs, and fish.
- **Vitamin K** is essential for bone formation and blood clotting; common food sources for vitamin K include leafy green vegetables.
- **Folic Acid** maintains healthy cells and blood and, when taken by a pregnant woman, can prevent her fetus from developing neural tube defects; food sources for folic acid include nuts, fortified breads, leafy green vegetables, and whole grains.

It should be noted that one can overdose on certain vitamins which become toxic if consumed in excess (e.g. vitamin A, D, E and K).

Like vitamins, minerals are chemicals that are required by the body to remain in good health. Because the human body does not manufacture these chemicals internally, we obtain them from food and other dietary sources. The more important minerals include:

- **Calcium** is needed for healthy bones, teeth, and muscles, but also helps the nervous system function; food sources for calcium include dry beans, peas, eggs, and dairy products.
- **Chromium** is helpful in regulating sugar levels in blood; food sources for chromium include egg yolks, raw sugar, cheese, nuts, beets, whole grains, and meat.

- **Fluoride** is used by the body to help prevent tooth decay and to reinforce bone strength; sources of fluoride include drinking water and certain brands of toothpaste.

- **Iodine** helps regulate the body's use of energy by synthesizing into the hormone thyroxine; food sources include leafy green vegetables, nuts, egg yolks, and red meat.

- **Iron** helps maintain muscles and the formation of red blood cells and certain proteins; food sources for iron include meat, dairy products, eggs, and leafy green vegetables.

- **Magnesium** is important for the production of DNA, as well as for healthy teeth, bones, muscles, and nerves; food sources for magnesium include dried fruit, dark green vegetables, nuts, and seafood.

- **Phosphorous** is used by the body to work with calcium to form bones and teeth; food sources for phosphorous include eggs, meat, cereals, and dairy products.

- **Selenium** primarily helps maintain normal heart and liver functions; food sources for selenium include wholegrain cereals, fish, meat, and dairy products.

- **Zinc** helps wounds heal, the formation of sperm, and encourage rapid growth and energy; food sources include dried beans, shellfish, eggs, and nuts.

The United States government periodically publishes recommended diets and consumption levels of the various elements of food. Again, your doctor may encourage deviations from the average official recommendation based on your specific condition. To learn more about basic dietary guidelines, visit the Web site: **http://www.health.gov/dietaryguidelines/**. Based on these guidelines, many foods are required to list the nutrition levels on the food's packaging. Labeling Requirements are listed at the following site maintained by the Food and Drug Administration: **http://www.cfsan.fda.gov/~dms/lab-cons.html**. When interpreting these requirements, the government recommends that consumers become familiar with the following abbreviations before reading FDA literature:[78]

- **DVs (Daily Values):** A new dietary reference term that will appear on the food label. It is made up of two sets of references, DRVs and RDIs.

- **DRVs (Daily Reference Values):** A set of dietary references that applies to fat, saturated fat, cholesterol, carbohydrate, protein, fiber, sodium, and potassium.

---

[78] Adapted from the FDA: **http://www.fda.gov/fdac/special/foodlabel/dvs.html**.

- **RDIs (Reference Daily Intakes):** A set of dietary references based on the Recommended Dietary Allowances for essential vitamins and minerals and, in selected groups, protein. The name "RDI" replaces the term "U.S. RDA."
- **RDAs (Recommended Dietary Allowances):** A set of estimated nutrient allowances established by the National Academy of Sciences. It is updated periodically to reflect current scientific knowledge.

What Are Dietary Supplements?[79]

Dietary supplements are widely available through many commercial sources, including health food stores, grocery stores, pharmacies, and by mail. Dietary supplements are provided in many forms including tablets, capsules, powders, gel-tabs, extracts, and liquids. Historically in the United States, the most prevalent type of dietary supplement was a multivitamin/mineral tablet or capsule that was available in pharmacies, either by prescription or "over the counter." Supplements containing strictly herbal preparations were less widely available. Currently in the United States, a wide array of supplement products are available, including vitamin, mineral, other nutrients, and botanical supplements as well as ingredients and extracts of animal and plant origin.

The Office of Dietary Supplements (ODS) of the National Institutes of Health is the official agency of the United States which has the expressed goal of acquiring "new knowledge to help prevent, detect, diagnose, and treat disease and disability, from the rarest genetic disorder to the common cold."[80] According to the ODS, dietary supplements can have an important impact on the prevention and management of disease and on the maintenance of health.[81] The ODS notes that considerable research on the effects of dietary supplements has been conducted in Asia and Europe where

---

[79] This discussion has been adapted from the NIH: **http://ods.od.nih.gov/whatare/whatare.html**.

[80] Contact: The Office of Dietary Supplements, National Institutes of Health, Building 31, Room 1B29, 31 Center Drive, MSC 2086, Bethesda, Maryland 20892-2086, Tel: (301) 435-2920, Fax: (301) 480-1845, E-mail: **ods@nih.gov**.

[81] Adapted from **http://ods.od.nih.gov/about/about.html**. The Dietary Supplement Health and Education Act defines dietary supplements as "a product (other than tobacco) intended to supplement the diet that bears or contains one or more of the following dietary ingredients: a vitamin, mineral, amino acid, herb or other botanical; or a dietary substance for use to supplement the diet by increasing the total dietary intake; or a concentrate, metabolite, constituent, extract, or combination of any ingredient described above; and intended for ingestion in the form of a capsule, powder, softgel, or gelcap, and not represented as a conventional food or as a sole item of a meal or the diet."

the use of plant products, in particular, has a long tradition. However, the overwhelming majority of supplements have not been studied scientifically. To explore the role of dietary supplements in the improvement of health care, the ODS plans, organizes, and supports conferences, workshops, and symposia on scientific topics related to dietary supplements. The ODS often works in conjunction with other NIH Institutes and Centers, other government agencies, professional organizations, and public advocacy groups.

To learn more about official information on dietary supplements, visit the ODS site at **http://ods.od.nih.gov/whatare/whatare.html**. Or contact:

> The Office of Dietary Supplements
> National Institutes of Health
> Building 31, Room 1B29
> 31 Center Drive, MSC 2086
> Bethesda, Maryland 20892-2086
> Tel: (301) 435-2920
> Fax: (301) 480-1845
> E-mail: ods@nih.gov

Finding Studies on Merkel Cell Carcinoma

The NIH maintains an office dedicated to patient nutrition and diet. The National Institutes of Health's Office of Dietary Supplements (ODS) offers a searchable bibliographic database called the IBIDS (International Bibliographic Information on Dietary Supplements). The IBIDS contains over 460,000 scientific citations and summaries about dietary supplements and nutrition as well as references to published international, scientific literature on dietary supplements such as vitamins, minerals, and botanicals.[82] IBIDS is available to the public free of charge through the ODS Internet page: **http://ods.od.nih.gov/databases/ibids.html**.

After entering the search area, you have three choices: (1) IBIDS Consumer Database, (2) Full IBIDS Database, or (3) Peer Reviewed Citations Only. We recommend that you start with the Consumer Database. While you may not find references for the topics that are of most interest to you, check back

---

[82] Adapted from **http://ods.od.nih.gov**. IBIDS is produced by the Office of Dietary Supplements (ODS) at the National Institutes of Health to assist the public, healthcare providers, educators, and researchers in locating credible, scientific information on dietary supplements. IBIDS was developed and will be maintained through an interagency partnership with the Food and Nutrition Information Center of the National Agricultural Library, U.S. Department of Agriculture.

periodically as this database is frequently updated. More studies can be found by searching the Full IBIDS Database. Healthcare professionals and researchers generally use the third option, which lists peer-reviewed citations. In all cases, we suggest that you take advantage of the "Advanced Search" option that allows you to retrieve up to 100 fully explained references in a comprehensive format. Type "merkel cell carcinoma" (or synonyms) into the search box. To narrow the search, you can also select the "Title" field.

The following information is typical of that found when using the "Full IBIDS Database" when searching using "merkel cell carcinoma" (or a synonym):

- **Analysis of toxicity of Merkel cell carcinoma of the skin treated with synchronous carboplatin/etoposide and radiation: a Trans-Tasman Radiation Oncology Group study.**
  Author(s): Division of Oncology Incorporating Queensland Radium Institute, Royal Brisbane Hospital, Herston, Queensland, Australia. M.Poulsen@mailbox.uq.edu.au
  Source: Poulsen, M Rischin, D Walpole, E Harvey, J Macintosh, J Ainslie, J Hamilton, C Keller, J Tripcony, L Int-J-Radiat-Oncol-Biol-Phys. 2001 September 1; 51(1): 156-63 0360-3016

- **Applicability of the sentinel node technique to Merkel cell carcinoma.**
  Author(s): Department of Surgery B, Rabin Medical Center, Beilinson Campus, Petach Tikva, Israel.
  Source: Wasserberg, N Schachter, J Fenig, E Feinmesser, M Gutman, H Dermatol-Surg. 2000 February; 26(2): 138-41 1076-0512

- **Chemotherapy for Merkel cell carcinoma with carboplatin and etoposide.**
  Author(s): 1st Department of Medical Oncology, Metaxas Memorial Cancer Hospital, Piraeus, Greece.
  Source: Pectasides, D Moutzourides, G Dimitriadis, M Varthalitis, J Athanassiou, A Am-J-Clin-Oncol. 1995 October; 18(5): 418-20 0277-3732

- **Chemotherapy of metastatic Merkel cell carcinoma: case report and review of the literature.**
  Author(s): Division of Medical Oncology, University of Southern California Comprehensive Cancer Center, Los Angeles 90033.
  Source: Sharma, D Flora, G Grunberg, S M Am-J-Clin-Oncol. 1991 April; 14(2): 166-9 0277-3732

- **Diagnostic pitfalls of Merkel cell carcinoma and dramatic response to chemotherapy.**
  Author(s): Department of Dermatology, Asan Medical Center, College of Medicine, University of Ulsan, Seoul, Korea.
  Source: Chang, S F Suh, J W Choi, J H Yoon, G S Huh, J Sung, K J Moon, K C Kim, W G Koh, J K J-Dermatol. 1998 May; 25(5): 322-8 0385-2407

- **Farnesylthiosalicylic acid inhibits the growth of human Merkel cell carcinoma in SCID mice.**
  Author(s): Department of Dermatology, University of Vienna, Austria.
  Source: Jansen, B Heere Ress, E Schlagbauer Wadl, H Halaschek Wiener, J Waltering, S Moll, I Pehamberger, H Marciano, D Kloog, Y Wolff, K J-Mol-Med. 1999 November; 77(11): 792-7 0946-2716

- **Lectin and proteoglycan histochemistry of Merkel cell carcinomas.**
  Author(s): Institut fur Anatomie, Universitatsklinikum Hamburg-Eppendorf, Martinistrasse 52, D-20246 Hamburg, Germany.
  Source: Sames, K Schumacher, U Halata, Z Van Damme, E J Peumans, W J Asmus, B Moll, R Moll, I Exp-Dermatol. 2001 April; 10(2): 100-9 0906-6705

- **Merkel cell carcinoma of the scalp: dramatic resolution with primary chemotherapy.**
  Author(s): Medical Oncology Unit USL 34, Catania, Italy.
  Source: Ferrau, F Micali, G Guitart, J J-Am-Acad-Dermatol. 1994 August; 31(2 Pt 1): 271-2 0190-9622

- **Neurologic complications of Merkel cell carcinoma.**
  Author(s): Department of Neurology, University Hospitals of Cleveland/Case Western Reserve School of Medicine, Ohio, USA.
  Source: Snodgrass, S M Landy, H Markoe, A M Feun, L J-Neurooncol. 1994; 22(3): 231-4 0167-594X

- **Oral etoposide for Merkel cell carcinoma in patients previously treated with intravenous etoposide.**
  Author(s): Institute of Oncology, Rabin Medical Center, Beilinson Campus, Petah Tiqva, Israel.
  Source: Fenig, E Brenner, B Njuguna, E Katz, A Schachter, J Sulkes, A Am-J-Clin-Oncol. 2000 February; 23(1): 65-7 0277-3732

- **The use of VP16 and cisplatin in the treatment of Merkel cell carcinoma.**
  Author(s): Riverside Regional Cancer Institute, Columbus, Ohio.
  Source: Davis, M P Miller, E M Rau, R C Johnson, O E Naille, R A Crnkovich, M J J-Dermatol-Surg-Oncol. 1990 March; 16(3): 276-8 0148-0812

- **Transient complete remission of metastasized Merkel cell carcinoma by high-dose polychemotherapy and autologous peripheral blood stem cell transplantation.**
  Author(s): Department of Dermatology, University of Heidelberg, Vossstr. 2, 69115 Heidelberg, Germany.
  Source: Waldmann, V Goldschmidt, H Jackel, A Deichmann, M Hegenbart, U Hartschuh, W Ho, A Naher, H Br-J-Dermatol. 2000 October; 143(4): 837-9 0007-0963

- **VP-16, cisplatin, doxorubicin, and bleomycin in metastatic Merkel cell carcinoma. Report of a case with long-term remission.**
  Author(s): Medical Oncology Service, Centre H. Becquerel, Rouen, France.
  Source: Azagury, M Chevallier, B Atlan, D Graic, Y Dayot, J P Thomine, E Am-J-Clin-Oncol. 1993 April; 16(2): 102-4 0277-3732

Federal Resources on Nutrition

In addition to the IBIDS, the United States Department of Health and Human Services (HHS) and the United States Department of Agriculture (USDA) provide many sources of information on general nutrition and health. Recommended resources include:

- healthfinder®, HHS's gateway to health information, including diet and nutrition:
  http://www.healthfinder.gov/scripts/SearchContext.asp?topic=238&page=0

- The United States Department of Agriculture's Web site dedicated to nutrition information: **www.nutrition.gov**

- The Food and Drug Administration's Web site for federal food safety information: **www.foodsafety.gov**

- The National Action Plan on Overweight and Obesity sponsored by the United States Surgeon General: **http://www.surgeongeneral.gov/topics/obesity/**

- The Center for Food Safety and Applied Nutrition has an Internet site sponsored by the Food and Drug Administration and the Department of Health and Human Services: **http://vm.cfsan.fda.gov/**

- Center for Nutrition Policy and Promotion sponsored by the United States Department of Agriculture: **http://www.usda.gov/cnpp/**

- Food and Nutrition Information Center, National Agricultural Library sponsored by the United States Department of Agriculture: **http://www.nal.usda.gov/fnic/**

- Food and Nutrition Service sponsored by the United States Department of Agriculture: http://www.fns.usda.gov/fns/

Additional Web Resources

A number of additional Web sites offer encyclopedic information covering food and nutrition. The following is a representative sample:

- AOL: http://search.aol.com/cat.adp?id=174&layer=&from=subcats
- Family Village: http://www.familyvillage.wisc.edu/med_nutrition.html
- Google: http://directory.google.com/Top/Health/Nutrition/
- Healthnotes: http://www.thedacare.org/healthnotes/
- Open Directory Project: http://dmoz.org/Health/Nutrition/
- Yahoo.com: http://dir.yahoo.com/Health/Nutrition/
- WebMD®Health: http://my.webmd.com/nutrition
- WholeHealthMD.com: http://www.wholehealthmd.com/reflib/0,1529,,00.html

Vocabulary Builder

The following vocabulary builder defines words used in the references in this chapter that have not been defined in previous chapters:

Bacteria: A large group of single-cell microorganisms. Some cause infections and disease in animals and humans. The singular of bacteria is bacterium. [NIH]

Calcium: A mineral found in teeth, bones, and other body tissues. [NIH]

Capsules: Hard or soft soluble containers used for the oral administration of medicine. [NIH]

Carbohydrate: An aldehyde or ketone derivative of a polyhydric alcohol, particularly of the pentahydric and hexahydric alcohols. They are so named because the hydrogen and oxygen are usually in the proportion to form water, $(CH2O)n$. The most important carbohydrates are the starches, sugars, celluloses, and gums. They are classified into mono-, di-, tri-, poly- and heterosaccharides. [EU]

Cholesterol: The principal sterol of all higher animals, distributed in body tissues, especially the brain and spinal cord, and in animal fats and oils. [NIH]

Diarrhea: Passage of excessively liquid or excessively frequent stools. [NIH]

Fetus: The developing offspring from 7 to 8 weeks after conception until birth. [NIH]

Niacin: Water-soluble vitamin of the B complex occurring in various animal and plant tissues. Required by the body for the formation of coenzymes NAD and NADP. Has pellagra-curative, vasodilating, and antilipemic properties. [NIH]

Overdose: 1. to administer an excessive dose. 2. an excessive dose. [EU]

Phosphorous: Having to do with or containing the element phosphorus. [NIH]

Potassium: A metallic element that is important in body functions such as regulation of blood pressure and of water content in cells, transmission of nerve impulses, digestion, muscle contraction, and heart beat. [NIH]

Riboflavin: Nutritional factor found in milk, eggs, malted barley, liver, kidney, heart, and leafy vegetables. The richest natural source is yeast. It occurs in the free form only in the retina of the eye, in whey, and in urine; its principal forms in tissues and cells are as FMN and FAD. [NIH]

Selenium: An essential dietary mineral. [NIH]

Thermoregulation: Heat regulation. [EU]

Thyroxine: An amino acid of the thyroid gland which exerts a stimulating effect on thyroid metabolism. [NIH]

APPENDIX D. FINDING MEDICAL LIBRARIES

Overview

At a medical library you can find medical texts and reference books, consumer health publications, specialty newspapers and magazines, as well as medical journals. In this appendix, we show you how to quickly find a medical library in your area.

Preparation

Before going to the library, highlight the references mentioned in this sourcebook that you find interesting. Focus on those items that are not available via the Internet, and ask the reference librarian for help with your search. He or she may know of additional resources that could be helpful to you. Most importantly, your local public library and medical libraries have Interlibrary Loan programs with the National Library of Medicine (NLM), one of the largest medical collections in the world. According to the NLM, most of the literature in the general and historical collections of the National Library of Medicine is available on interlibrary loan to any library. NLM's interlibrary loan services are only available to libraries. If you would like to access NLM medical literature, then visit a library in your area that can request the publications for you.[83]

---

[83] Adapted from the NLM: http://www.nlm.nih.gov/psd/cas/interlibrary.html

Finding a Local Medical Library

The quickest method to locate medical libraries is to use the Internet-based directory published by the National Network of Libraries of Medicine (NN/LM). This network includes 4626 members and affiliates that provide many services to librarians, health professionals, and the public. To find a library in your area, simply visit **http://nnlm.gov/members/adv.html** or call 1-800-338-7657.

Medical Libraries Open to the Public

In addition to the NN/LM, the National Library of Medicine (NLM) lists a number of libraries that are generally open to the public and have reference facilities. The following is the NLM's list plus hyperlinks to each library Web site. These Web pages can provide information on hours of operation and other restrictions. The list below is a small sample of libraries recommended by the National Library of Medicine (sorted alphabetically by name of the U.S. state or Canadian province where the library is located):[84]

- **Alabama:** Health InfoNet of Jefferson County (Jefferson County Library Cooperative, Lister Hill Library of the Health Sciences), **http://www.uab.edu/infonet/**

- **Alabama:** Richard M. Scrushy Library (American Sports Medicine Institute), **http://www.asmi.org/LIBRARY.HTM**

- **Arizona:** Samaritan Regional Medical Center: The Learning Center (Samaritan Health System, Phoenix, Arizona), **http://www.samaritan.edu/library/bannerlibs.htm**

- **California:** Kris Kelly Health Information Center (St. Joseph Health System), **http://www.humboldt1.com/~kkhic/index.html**

- **California:** Community Health Library of Los Gatos (Community Health Library of Los Gatos), **http://www.healthlib.org/orgresources.html**

- **California:** Consumer Health Program and Services (CHIPS) (County of Los Angeles Public Library, Los Angeles County Harbor-UCLA Medical Center Library) - Carson, CA, **http://www.colapublib.org/services/chips.html**

- **California:** Gateway Health Library (Sutter Gould Medical Foundation)

- **California:** Health Library (Stanford University Medical Center), **http://www-med.stanford.edu/healthlibrary/**

---

[84] Abstracted from **http://www.nlm.nih.gov/medlineplus/libraries.html**.

- **California:** Patient Education Resource Center - Health Information and Resources (University of California, San Francisco), **http://sfghdean.ucsf.edu/barnett/PERC/default.asp**
- **California:** Redwood Health Library (Petaluma Health Care District), **http://www.phcd.org/rdwdlib.html**
- **California:** San José PlaneTree Health Library, **http://planetreesanjose.org/**
- **California:** Sutter Resource Library (Sutter Hospitals Foundation), **http://go.sutterhealth.org/comm/resc-library/sac-resources.html**
- **California:** University of California, Davis. Health Sciences Libraries
- **California:** ValleyCare Health Library & Ryan Comer Cancer Resource Center (ValleyCare Health System), **http://www.valleycare.com/library.html**
- **California:** Washington Community Health Resource Library (Washington Community Health Resource Library), **http://www.healthlibrary.org/**
- **Colorado:** William V. Gervasini Memorial Library (Exempla Healthcare), **http://www.exempla.org/conslib.htm**
- **Connecticut:** Hartford Hospital Health Science Libraries (Hartford Hospital), **http://www.harthosp.org/library/**
- **Connecticut:** Healthnet: Connecticut Consumer Health Information Center (University of Connecticut Health Center, Lyman Maynard Stowe Library), **http://library.uchc.edu/departm/hnet/**
- **Connecticut:** Waterbury Hospital Health Center Library (Waterbury Hospital), **http://www.waterburyhospital.com/library/consumer.shtml**
- **Delaware:** Consumer Health Library (Christiana Care Health System, Eugene du Pont Preventive Medicine & Rehabilitation Institute), **http://www.christianacare.org/health_guide/health_guide_pmri_health_info.cfm**
- **Delaware:** Lewis B. Flinn Library (Delaware Academy of Medicine), **http://www.delamed.org/chls.html**
- **Georgia:** Family Resource Library (Medical College of Georgia), **http://cmc.mcg.edu/kids_families/fam_resources/fam_res_lib/frl.htm**
- **Georgia:** Health Resource Center (Medical Center of Central Georgia), **http://www.mccg.org/hrc/hrchome.asp**
- **Hawaii:** Hawaii Medical Library: Consumer Health Information Service (Hawaii Medical Library), **http://hml.org/CHIS/**

- **Idaho:** DeArmond Consumer Health Library (Kootenai Medical Center), http://www.nicon.org/DeArmond/index.htm
- **Illinois:** Health Learning Center of Northwestern Memorial Hospital (Northwestern Memorial Hospital, Health Learning Center), http://www.nmh.org/health_info/hlc.html
- **Illinois:** Medical Library (OSF Saint Francis Medical Center), http://www.osfsaintfrancis.org/general/library/
- **Kentucky:** Medical Library - Services for Patients, Families, Students & the Public (Central Baptist Hospital), http://www.centralbap.com/education/community/library.htm
- **Kentucky:** University of Kentucky - Health Information Library (University of Kentucky, Chandler Medical Center, Health Information Library), http://www.mc.uky.edu/PatientEd/
- **Louisiana:** Alton Ochsner Medical Foundation Library (Alton Ochsner Medical Foundation), http://www.ochsner.org/library/
- **Louisiana:** Louisiana State University Health Sciences Center Medical Library-Shreveport, http://lib-sh.lsuhsc.edu/
- **Maine:** Franklin Memorial Hospital Medical Library (Franklin Memorial Hospital), http://www.fchn.org/fmh/lib.htm
- **Maine:** Gerrish-True Health Sciences Library (Central Maine Medical Center), http://www.cmmc.org/library/library.html
- **Maine:** Hadley Parrot Health Science Library (Eastern Maine Healthcare), http://www.emh.org/hll/hpl/guide.htm
- **Maine:** Maine Medical Center Library (Maine Medical Center), http://www.mmc.org/library/
- **Maine:** Parkview Hospital, http://www.parkviewhospital.org/communit.htm#Library
- **Maine:** Southern Maine Medical Center Health Sciences Library (Southern Maine Medical Center), http://www.smmc.org/services/service.php3?choice=10
- **Maine:** Stephens Memorial Hospital Health Information Library (Western Maine Health), http://www.wmhcc.com/hil_frame.html
- **Manitoba, Canada:** Consumer & Patient Health Information Service (University of Manitoba Libraries), http://www.umanitoba.ca/libraries/units/health/reference/chis.html
- **Manitoba, Canada:** J.W. Crane Memorial Library (Deer Lodge Centre), http://www.deerlodge.mb.ca/library/libraryservices.shtml

- **Maryland:** Health Information Center at the Wheaton Regional Library (Montgomery County, Md., Dept. of Public Libraries, Wheaton Regional Library), **http://www.mont.lib.md.us/healthinfo/hic.asp**
- **Massachusetts:** Baystate Medical Center Library (Baystate Health System), **http://www.baystatehealth.com/1024/**
- **Massachusetts:** Boston University Medical Center Alumni Medical Library (Boston University Medical Center), **http://med-libwww.bu.edu/library/lib.html**
- **Massachusetts:** Lowell General Hospital Health Sciences Library (Lowell General Hospital), **http://www.lowellgeneral.org/library/HomePageLinks/WWW.htm**
- **Massachusetts:** Paul E. Woodard Health Sciences Library (New England Baptist Hospital), **http://www.nebh.org/health_lib.asp**
- **Massachusetts:** St. Luke's Hospital Health Sciences Library (St. Luke's Hospital), **http://www.southcoast.org/library/**
- **Massachusetts:** Treadwell Library Consumer Health Reference Center (Massachusetts General Hospital), **http://www.mgh.harvard.edu/library/chrcindex.html**
- **Massachusetts:** UMass HealthNet (University of Massachusetts Medical School), **http://healthnet.umassmed.edu/**
- **Michigan:** Botsford General Hospital Library - Consumer Health (Botsford General Hospital, Library & Internet Services), **http://www.botsfordlibrary.org/consumer.htm**
- **Michigan:** Helen DeRoy Medical Library (Providence Hospital and Medical Centers), **http://www.providence-hospital.org/library/**
- **Michigan:** Marquette General Hospital - Consumer Health Library (Marquette General Hospital, Health Information Center), **http://www.mgh.org/center.html**
- **Michigan:** Patient Education Resouce Center - University of Michigan Cancer Center (University of Michigan Comprehensive Cancer Center), **http://www.cancer.med.umich.edu/learn/leares.htm**
- **Michigan:** Sladen Library & Center for Health Information Resources - Consumer Health Information, **http://www.sladen.hfhs.org/library/consumer/index.html**
- **Montana:** Center for Health Information (St. Patrick Hospital and Health Sciences Center), **http://www.saintpatrick.org/chi/librarydetail.php3?ID=41**

- **National:** Consumer Health Library Directory (Medical Library Association, Consumer and Patient Health Information Section), http://caphis.mlanet.org/directory/index.html
- **National:** National Network of Libraries of Medicine (National Library of Medicine) - provides library services for health professionals in the United States who do not have access to a medical library, http://nnlm.gov/
- **National:** NN/LM List of Libraries Serving the Public (National Network of Libraries of Medicine), http://nnlm.gov/members/
- **Nevada:** Health Science Library, West Charleston Library (Las Vegas Clark County Library District), http://www.lvccld.org/special_collections/medical/index.htm
- **New Hampshire:** Dartmouth Biomedical Libraries (Dartmouth College Library), http://www.dartmouth.edu/~biomed/resources.htmld/conshealth.htmld/
- **New Jersey:** Consumer Health Library (Rahway Hospital), http://www.rahwayhospital.com/library.htm
- **New Jersey:** Dr. Walter Phillips Health Sciences Library (Englewood Hospital and Medical Center), http://www.englewoodhospital.com/links/index.htm
- **New Jersey:** Meland Foundation (Englewood Hospital and Medical Center), http://www.geocities.com/ResearchTriangle/9360/
- **New York:** Choices in Health Information (New York Public Library) - NLM Consumer Pilot Project participant, http://www.nypl.org/branch/health/links.html
- **New York:** Health Information Center (Upstate Medical University, State University of New York), http://www.upstate.edu/library/hic/
- **New York:** Health Sciences Library (Long Island Jewish Medical Center), http://www.lij.edu/library/library.html
- **New York:** ViaHealth Medical Library (Rochester General Hospital), http://www.nyam.org/library/
- **Ohio:** Consumer Health Library (Akron General Medical Center, Medical & Consumer Health Library), http://www.akrongeneral.org/hwlibrary.htm
- **Oklahoma:** Saint Francis Health System Patient/Family Resource Center (Saint Francis Health System), http://www.sfh-tulsa.com/patientfamilycenter/default.asp

- **Oregon:** Planetree Health Resource Center (Mid-Columbia Medical Center), **http://www.mcmc.net/phrc/**
- **Pennsylvania:** Community Health Information Library (Milton S. Hershey Medical Center), **http://www.hmc.psu.edu/commhealth/**
- **Pennsylvania:** Community Health Resource Library (Geisinger Medical Center), **http://www.geisinger.edu/education/commlib.shtml**
- **Pennsylvania:** HealthInfo Library (Moses Taylor Hospital), **http://www.mth.org/healthwellness.html**
- **Pennsylvania:** Hopwood Library (University of Pittsburgh, Health Sciences Library System), **http://www.hsls.pitt.edu/chi/hhrcinfo.html**
- **Pennsylvania:** Koop Community Health Information Center (College of Physicians of Philadelphia), **http://www.collphyphil.org/kooppg1.shtml**
- **Pennsylvania:** Learning Resources Center - Medical Library (Susquehanna Health System), **http://www.shscares.org/services/lrc/index.asp**
- **Pennsylvania:** Medical Library (UPMC Health System), **http://www.upmc.edu/passavant/library.htm**
- **Quebec, Canada:** Medical Library (Montreal General Hospital), **http://ww2.mcgill.ca/mghlib/**
- **South Dakota:** Rapid City Regional Hospital - Health Information Center (Rapid City Regional Hospital, Health Information Center), **http://www.rcrh.org/education/LibraryResourcesConsumers.htm**
- **Texas:** Houston HealthWays (Houston Academy of Medicine-Texas Medical Center Library), **http://hhw.library.tmc.edu/**
- **Texas:** Matustik Family Resource Center (Cook Children's Health Care System), **http://www.cookchildrens.com/Matustik_Library.html**
- **Washington:** Community Health Library (Kittitas Valley Community Hospital), **http://www.kvch.com/**
- **Washington:** Southwest Washington Medical Center Library (Southwest Washington Medical Center), **http://www.swmedctr.com/Home/**

APPENDIX E. YOUR RIGHTS AND INSURANCE

Overview

Any patient with merkel cell carcinoma faces a series of issues related more to the healthcare industry than to the medical condition itself. This appendix covers two important topics in this regard: your rights and responsibilities as a patient, and how to get the most out of your medical insurance plan.

Your Rights as a Patient

The President's Advisory Commission on Consumer Protection and Quality in the Healthcare Industry has created the following summary of your rights as a patient.[85]

Information Disclosure

Consumers have the right to receive accurate, easily understood information. Some consumers require assistance in making informed decisions about health plans, health professionals, and healthcare facilities. Such information includes:

- *Health plans.* Covered benefits, cost-sharing, and procedures for resolving complaints, licensure, certification, and accreditation status, comparable measures of quality and consumer satisfaction, provider network composition, the procedures that govern access to specialists and emergency services, and care management information.

---

[85] Adapted from Consumer Bill of Rights and Responsibilities: **http://www.hcqualitycommission.gov/press/cbor.html#head1**.

- *Health professionals.* Education, board certification, and recertification, years of practice, experience performing certain procedures, and comparable measures of quality and consumer satisfaction.

- *Healthcare facilities.* Experience in performing certain procedures and services, accreditation status, comparable measures of quality, worker, and consumer satisfaction, and procedures for resolving complaints.

- *Consumer assistance programs.* Programs must be carefully structured to promote consumer confidence and to work cooperatively with health plans, providers, payers, and regulators. Desirable characteristics of such programs are sponsorship that ensures accountability to the interests of consumers and stable, adequate funding.

Choice of Providers and Plans

Consumers have the right to a choice of healthcare providers that is sufficient to ensure access to appropriate high-quality healthcare. To ensure such choice, the Commission recommends the following:

- *Provider network adequacy.* All health plan networks should provide access to sufficient numbers and types of providers to assure that all covered services will be accessible without unreasonable delay -- including access to emergency services 24 hours a day and 7 days a week. If a health plan has an insufficient number or type of providers to provide a covered benefit with the appropriate degree of specialization, the plan should ensure that the consumer obtains the benefit outside the network at no greater cost than if the benefit were obtained from participating providers.

- *Women's health services.* Women should be able to choose a qualified provider offered by a plan -- such as gynecologists, certified nurse midwives, and other qualified healthcare providers -- for the provision of covered care necessary to provide routine and preventative women's healthcare services.

- *Access to specialists.* Consumers with complex or serious medical conditions who require frequent specialty care should have direct access to a qualified specialist of their choice within a plan's network of providers. Authorizations, when required, should be for an adequate number of direct access visits under an approved treatment plan.

- *Transitional care.* Consumers who are undergoing a course of treatment for a chronic or disabling condition (or who are in the second or third trimester of a pregnancy) at the time they involuntarily change health plans or at a time when a provider is terminated by a plan for other than cause should be able to continue seeing their current specialty providers for up to 90 days (or through completion of postpartum care) to allow for transition of care.

- *Choice of health plans.* Public and private group purchasers should, wherever feasible, offer consumers a choice of high-quality health insurance plans.

Access to Emergency Services

Consumers have the right to access emergency healthcare services when and where the need arises. Health plans should provide payment when a consumer presents to an emergency department with acute symptoms of sufficient severity--including severe pain--such that a "prudent layperson" could reasonably expect the absence of medical attention to result in placing that consumer's health in serious jeopardy, serious impairment to bodily functions, or serious dysfunction of any bodily organ or part.

Participation in Treatment Decisions

Consumers have the right and responsibility to fully participate in all decisions related to their healthcare. Consumers who are unable to fully participate in treatment decisions have the right to be represented by parents, guardians, family members, or other conservators. Physicians and other health professionals should:

- Provide patients with sufficient information and opportunity to decide among treatment options consistent with the informed consent process.
- Discuss all treatment options with a patient in a culturally competent manner, including the option of no treatment at all.
- Ensure that persons with disabilities have effective communications with members of the health system in making such decisions.
- Discuss all current treatments a consumer may be undergoing.
- Discuss all risks, benefits, and consequences to treatment or nontreatment.
- Give patients the opportunity to refuse treatment and to express preferences about future treatment decisions.

- Discuss the use of advance directives -- both living wills and durable powers of attorney for healthcare -- with patients and their designated family members.

- Abide by the decisions made by their patients and/or their designated representatives consistent with the informed consent process.

Health plans, health providers, and healthcare facilities should:

- Disclose to consumers factors -- such as methods of compensation, ownership of or interest in healthcare facilities, or matters of conscience -- that could influence advice or treatment decisions.

- Assure that provider contracts do not contain any so-called "gag clauses" or other contractual mechanisms that restrict healthcare providers' ability to communicate with and advise patients about medically necessary treatment options.

- Be prohibited from penalizing or seeking retribution against healthcare professionals or other health workers for advocating on behalf of their patients.

Respect and Nondiscrimination

Consumers have the right to considerate, respectful care from all members of the healthcare industry at all times and under all circumstances. An environment of mutual respect is essential to maintain a quality healthcare system. To assure that right, the Commission recommends the following:

- Consumers must not be discriminated against in the delivery of healthcare services consistent with the benefits covered in their policy, or as required by law, based on race, ethnicity, national origin, religion, sex, age, mental or physical disability, sexual orientation, genetic information, or source of payment.

- Consumers eligible for coverage under the terms and conditions of a health plan or program, or as required by law, must not be discriminated against in marketing and enrollment practices based on race, ethnicity, national origin, religion, sex, age, mental or physical disability, sexual orientation, genetic information, or source of payment.

Confidentiality of Health Information

Consumers have the right to communicate with healthcare providers in confidence and to have the confidentiality of their individually identifiable healthcare information protected. Consumers also have the right to review and copy their own medical records and request amendments to their records.

Complaints and Appeals

Consumers have the right to a fair and efficient process for resolving differences with their health plans, healthcare providers, and the institutions that serve them, including a rigorous system of internal review and an independent system of external review. A free copy of the Patient's Bill of Rights is available from the American Hospital Association.[86]

Patient Responsibilities

Treatment is a two-way street between you and your healthcare providers. To underscore the importance of finance in modern healthcare as well as your responsibility for the financial aspects of your care, the President's Advisory Commission on Consumer Protection and Quality in the Healthcare Industry has proposed that patients understand the following "Consumer Responsibilities."[87] In a healthcare system that protects consumers' rights, it is reasonable to expect and encourage consumers to assume certain responsibilities. Greater individual involvement by the consumer in his or her care increases the likelihood of achieving the best outcome and helps support a quality-oriented, cost-conscious environment. Such responsibilities include:

- Take responsibility for maximizing healthy habits such as exercising, not smoking, and eating a healthy diet.
- Work collaboratively with healthcare providers in developing and carrying out agreed-upon treatment plans.
- Disclose relevant information and clearly communicate wants and needs.
- Use your health insurance plan's internal complaint and appeal processes to address your concerns.
- Avoid knowingly spreading disease.

---

[86] To order your free copy of the Patient's Bill of Rights, telephone 312-422-3000 or visit the American Hospital Association's Web site: **http://www.aha.org**. Click on "Resource Center," go to "Search" at bottom of page, and then type in "Patient's Bill of Rights." The Patient's Bill of Rights is also available from Fax on Demand, at 312-422-2020, document number 471124.

[87] Adapted from **http://www.hcqualitycommission.gov/press/cbor.html#head1**.

- Recognize the reality of risks, the limits of the medical science, and the human fallibility of the healthcare professional.

- Be aware of a healthcare provider's obligation to be reasonably efficient and equitable in providing care to other patients and the community.

- Become knowledgeable about your health plan's coverage and options (when available) including all covered benefits, limitations, and exclusions, rules regarding use of network providers, coverage and referral rules, appropriate processes to secure additional information, and the process to appeal coverage decisions.

- Show respect for other patients and health workers.

- Make a good-faith effort to meet financial obligations.

- Abide by administrative and operational procedures of health plans, healthcare providers, and Government health benefit programs.

Choosing an Insurance Plan

There are a number of official government agencies that help consumers understand their healthcare insurance choices.[88] The U.S. Department of Labor, in particular, recommends ten ways to make your health benefits choices work best for you.[89]

1. Your options are important. There are many different types of health benefit plans. Find out which one your employer offers, then check out the plan, or plans, offered. Your employer's human resource office, the health plan administrator, or your union can provide information to help you match your needs and preferences with the available plans. The more information you have, the better your healthcare decisions will be.

2. Reviewing the benefits available. Do the plans offered cover preventive care, well-baby care, vision or dental care? Are there deductibles? Answers to these questions can help determine the out-of-pocket expenses you may face. Matching your needs and those of your family members will result in the best possible benefits. Cheapest may not always be best. Your goal is high quality health benefits.

---

[88] More information about quality across programs is provided at the following AHRQ Web site:
http://www.ahrq.gov/consumer/qntascii/qnthplan.htm .
[89] Adapted from the Department of Labor:
http://www.dol.gov/dol/pwba/public/pubs/health/top10-text.html.

3. Look for quality. The quality of healthcare services varies, but quality can be measured. You should consider the quality of healthcare in deciding among the healthcare plans or options available to you. Not all health plans, doctors, hospitals and other providers give the highest quality care. Fortunately, there is quality information you can use right now to help you compare your healthcare choices. Find out how you can measure quality. Consult the U.S. Department of Health and Human Services publication "Your Guide to Choosing Quality Health Care" on the Internet at **www.ahcpr.gov/consumer**.

4. Your plan's summary plan description (SPD) provides a wealth of information. Your health plan administrator can provide you with a copy of your plan's SPD. It outlines your benefits and your legal rights under the Employee Retirement Income Security Act (ERISA), the federal law that protects your health benefits. It should contain information about the coverage of dependents, what services will require a co-pay, and the circumstances under which your employer can change or terminate a health benefits plan. Save the SPD and all other health plan brochures and documents, along with memos or correspondence from your employer relating to health benefits.

5. Assess your benefit coverage as your family status changes. Marriage, divorce, childbirth or adoption, and the death of a spouse are all life events that may signal a need to change your health benefits. You, your spouse and dependent children may be eligible for a special enrollment period under provisions of the Health Insurance Portability and Accountability Act (HIPAA). Even without life-changing events, the information provided by your employer should tell you how you can change benefits or switch plans, if more than one plan is offered. If your spouse's employer also offers a health benefits package, consider coordinating both plans for maximum coverage.

6. Changing jobs and other life events can affect your health benefits. Under the Consolidated Omnibus Budget Reconciliation Act (COBRA), you, your covered spouse, and your dependent children may be eligible to purchase extended health coverage under your employer's plan if you lose your job, change employers, get divorced, or upon occurrence of certain other events. Coverage can range from 18 to 36 months depending on your situation. COBRA applies to most employers with 20 or more workers and requires your plan to notify you of your rights. Most plans require eligible individuals to make their COBRA election within 60 days of the plan's notice. Be sure to follow up with your plan sponsor if you don't receive notice, and make sure you respond within the allotted time.

7. HIPAA can also help if you are changing jobs, particularly if you have a medical condition. HIPAA generally limits pre-existing condition exclusions to a maximum of 12 months (18 months for late enrollees). HIPAA also requires this maximum period to be reduced by the length of time you had prior "creditable coverage." You should receive a certificate documenting your prior creditable coverage from your old plan when coverage ends.

8. Plan for retirement. Before you retire, find out what health benefits, if any, extend to you and your spouse during your retirement years. Consult with your employer's human resources office, your union, the plan administrator, and check your SPD. Make sure there is no conflicting information among these sources about the benefits you will receive or the circumstances under which they can change or be eliminated. With this information in hand, you can make other important choices, like finding out if you are eligible for Medicare and Medigap insurance coverage.

9. Know how to file an appeal if your health benefits claim is denied. Understand how your plan handles grievances and where to make appeals of the plan's decisions. Keep records and copies of correspondence. Check your health benefits package and your SPD to determine who is responsible for handling problems with benefit claims. Contact PWBA for customer service assistance if you are unable to obtain a response to your complaint.

10. You can take steps to improve the quality of the healthcare and the health benefits you receive. Look for and use things like Quality Reports and Accreditation Reports whenever you can. Quality reports may contain consumer ratings -- how satisfied consumers are with the doctors in their plan, for instance-- and clinical performance measures -- how well a healthcare organization prevents and treats illness. Accreditation reports provide information on how accredited organizations meet national standards, and often include clinical performance measures. Look for these quality measures whenever possible. Consult "Your Guide to Choosing Quality Health Care" on the Internet at **www.ahcpr.gov/consumer**.

Medicare and Medicaid

Illness strikes both rich and poor families. For low-income families, Medicaid is available to defer the costs of treatment. The Health Care Financing Administration (HCFA) administers Medicare, the nation's largest health insurance program, which covers 39 million Americans. In the following pages, you will learn the basics about Medicare insurance as well as useful contact information on how to find more in-depth information about Medicaid.[90]

Who is Eligible for Medicare?

Generally, you are eligible for Medicare if you or your spouse worked for at least 10 years in Medicare-covered employment and you are 65 years old and a citizen or permanent resident of the United States. You might also qualify for coverage if you are under age 65 but have a disability or End-Stage Renal disease (permanent kidney failure requiring dialysis or transplant). Here are some simple guidelines:

You can get Part A at age 65 without having to pay premiums if:

- You are already receiving retirement benefits from Social Security or the Railroad Retirement Board.
- You are eligible to receive Social Security or Railroad benefits but have not yet filed for them.
- You or your spouse had Medicare-covered government employment.

If you are under 65, you can get Part A without having to pay premiums if:

- You have received Social Security or Railroad Retirement Board disability benefit for 24 months.
- You are a kidney dialysis or kidney transplant patient.

Medicare has two parts:
- Part A (Hospital Insurance). Most people do not have to pay for Part A.
- Part B (Medical Insurance). Most people pay monthly for Part B.

Part A (Hospital Insurance)

Helps Pay For: Inpatient hospital care, care in critical access hospitals (small facilities that give limited outpatient and inpatient services to people in rural areas) and skilled nursing facilities, hospice care, and some home healthcare.

---

[90] This section has been adapted from the Official U.S. Site for Medicare Information: **http://www.medicare.gov/Basics/Overview.asp**.

Cost: Most people get Part A automatically when they turn age 65. You do not have to pay a monthly payment called a premium for Part A because you or a spouse paid Medicare taxes while you were working.

If you (or your spouse) did not pay Medicare taxes while you were working and you are age 65 or older, you still may be able to buy Part A. If you are not sure you have Part A, look on your red, white, and blue Medicare card. It will show "Hospital Part A" on the lower left corner of the card. You can also call the Social Security Administration toll free at 1-800-772-1213 or call your local Social Security office for more information about buying Part A. If you get benefits from the Railroad Retirement Board, call your local RRB office or 1-800-808-0772. For more information, call your Fiscal Intermediary about Part A bills and services. The phone number for the Fiscal Intermediary office in your area can be obtained from the following Web site: **http://www.medicare.gov/Contacts/home.asp**.

Part B (Medical Insurance)

Helps Pay For: Doctors, services, outpatient hospital care, and some other medical services that Part A does not cover, such as the services of physical and occupational therapists, and some home healthcare. Part B helps pay for covered services and supplies when they are medically necessary.

Cost: As of 2001, you pay the Medicare Part B premium of $50.00 per month. In some cases this amount may be higher if you did not choose Part B when you first became eligible at age 65. The cost of Part B may go up 10% for each 12-month period that you were eligible for Part B but declined coverage, except in special cases. You will have to pay the extra 10% cost for the rest of your life.

Enrolling in Part B is your choice. You can sign up for Part B anytime during a 7-month period that begins 3 months before you turn 65. Visit your local Social Security office, or call the Social Security Administration at 1-800-772-1213 to sign up. If you choose to enroll in Part B, the premium is usually taken out of your monthly Social Security, Railroad Retirement, or Civil Service Retirement payment. If you do not receive any of the above payments, Medicare sends you a bill for your part B premium every 3 months. You should receive your Medicare premium bill in the mail by the 10th of the month. If you do not, call the Social Security Administration at 1-800-772-1213, or your local Social Security office. If you get benefits from the Railroad Retirement Board, call your local RRB office or 1-800-808-0772. For more information, call your Medicare carrier about bills and services. The phone number for the Medicare carrier in your area can be found at the following Web site: **http://www.medicare.gov/Contacts/home.asp**. You may have choices in how you get your healthcare including the Original Medicare Plan, Medicare Managed Care Plans (like HMOs), and Medicare Private Fee-for-Service Plans.

Medicaid

Medicaid is a joint federal and state program that helps pay medical costs for some people with low incomes and limited resources. Medicaid programs vary from state to state. People on Medicaid may also get coverage for nursing home care and outpatient prescription drugs which are not covered by Medicare. You can find more information about Medicaid on the HCFA.gov Web site at **http://www.hcfa.gov/medicaid/medicaid.htm**.

States also have programs that pay some or all of Medicare's premiums and may also pay Medicare deductibles and coinsurance for certain people who have Medicare and a low income. To qualify, you must have:

- Part A (Hospital Insurance),
- Assets, such as bank accounts, stocks, and bonds that are not more than $4,000 for a single person, or $6,000 for a couple, and
- A monthly income that is below certain limits.

For more information on these programs, look at the Medicare Savings Programs brochure, **http://www.medicare.gov/Library/PDFNavigation/PDFInterim.asp?Language=English&Type=Pub&PubID=10126**. There are also Prescription Drug Assistance Programs available. Find information on these programs which offer discounts or free medications to individuals in need at **http://www.medicare.gov/Prescription/Home.asp**.

Financial Assistance for Cancer Care[91]

Cancer imposes heavy economic burdens on both patients and their families. For many people, a portion of medical expenses is paid by their health insurance plan. For individuals who do not have health insurance or who need financial assistance to cover health care costs, resources are available,

---

[91] Adapted from the NCI: **http://cis.nci.nih.gov/fact/8_3.htm**.

including government-sponsored programs and services supported by voluntary organizations.

Cancer patients and their families should discuss any concerns they may have about health care costs with their physician, medical social worker, or the business office of their hospital or clinic.

The organizations and resources listed below may offer financial assistance. Organizations that provide publications in Spanish or have Spanish-speaking staff have been identified.

- The American Cancer Society (ACS) office can provide the telephone number of the local ACS office serving your area. The local ACS office may offer reimbursement for expenses related to cancer treatment including transportation, medicine, and medical supplies. The ACS also offers programs that help cancer patients, family members, and friends cope with the emotional challenges they face. Some publications are available in Spanish. Spanish-speaking staff are available. Telephone: 1-800-ACS-2345 (1-800-227-2345). Web site: **http://www.cancer.org**

- The *AVONCares* Program for Medically Underserved Women provides financial assistance and relevant education and support to low income, under- and uninsured, underserved women throughout the country in need of diagnostic and/or related services (transportation, child care, and social support) for the treatment of breast, cervical, and ovarian cancers. Telephone: 1-800-813-HOPE (1-800-813-4673). Web site: **http://www.cancercare.org**.

Community voluntary agencies and service organizations such as the Salvation Army, Lutheran Social Services, Jewish Social Services, Catholic Charities, and the Lions Club may offer help. These organizations are listed in your local phone directory. Some churches and synagogues may provide financial help or services to their members.
Fundraising is another mechanism to consider. Some patients find that friends, family, and community members are willing to contribute financially if they are aware of a difficult situation. Contact your local library for information about how to organize fundraising efforts.

General assistance programs provide food, housing, prescription drugs, and other medical expenses for those who are not eligible for other programs. Funds are often limited. Information can be obtained by contacting your state or local Department of Social Services; this number is found in the local telephone directory.

Hill-Burton is a program through which hospitals receive construction funds from the Federal Government. Hospitals that receive Hill-Burton funds are required by law to provide some services to people who cannot afford to pay for their hospitalization. Information about which facilities are part of this program is available by calling the toll-free number or visiting the Web site shown below. A brochure about the program is available in Spanish. Telephone: 1-800-638-0742. Web site: **http://www.hrsa.gov/osp/dfcr/obtain/consfaq.htm**.

Income Tax Deductions

Medical costs that are not covered by insurance policies sometimes can be deducted from annual income before taxes. Examples of tax deductible expenses might include mileage for trips to and from medical appointments, out-of-pocket costs for treatment, prescription drugs or equipment, and the cost of meals during lengthy medical visits. The local Internal Revenue Service office, tax consultants, or certified public accountants can determine medical costs that are tax deductible. These telephone numbers are available in the local telephone directory. Web site: **http://www.irs.ustreas.gov**.

The Patient Advocate Foundation

The Patient Advocate Foundation (PAF) is a national nonprofit organization that provides education, legal counseling, and referrals to cancer patients and survivors concerning managed care, insurance, financial issues, job discrimination, and debt crisis matters. Telephone: 1-800-532-5274. **Web site: http://www.patientadvocate.org**.

Patient Assistance Programs are offered by some pharmaceutical manufacturers to help pay for medications. To learn whether a specific drug might be available at reduced cost through such a program, talk with a physician or a medical social worker.

Transportation

There are nonprofit organizations that arrange free or reduced cost air transportation for cancer patients going to or from cancer treatment centers. Financial need is not always a requirement. To find out about these programs, talk with a medical social worker. Ground transportation services may be offered or mileage reimbursed through the local ACS or your state or local Department of Social Services.

Veterans Benefits

Eligible veterans and their dependents may receive cancer treatment at a Veterans Administration Medical Center. Treatment for service-connected conditions is provided, and treatment for other conditions may be available based on the veteran's financial need. Some publications are available in Spanish. Spanish-speaking staff are available in some offices. Telephone: 1-877-222-VETS. Web site: **http://www.va.gov/vbs/health**.

NORD's Medication Assistance Programs

Finally, the National Organization for Rare Disorders, Inc. (NORD) administers medication programs sponsored by humanitarian-minded pharmaceutical and biotechnology companies to help uninsured or under-insured individuals secure life-saving or life-sustaining drugs.[92] NORD programs ensure that certain vital drugs are available "to those individuals whose income is too high to qualify for Medicaid but too low to pay for their prescribed medications." The program has standards for fairness, equity, and unbiased eligibility. It currently covers some 14 programs for nine pharmaceutical companies. NORD also offers early access programs for investigational new drugs (IND) under the approved "Treatment INDs" programs of the Food and Drug Administration (FDA). In these programs, a limited number of individuals can receive investigational drugs that have yet to be approved by the FDA. These programs are generally designed for rare diseases or disorders. For more information, visit **www.rarediseases.org**.

---

[92] Adapted from NORD: **http://www.rarediseases.org/cgi-bin/nord/progserv#patient?id=rPIzL9oD&mv_pc=30**.

Additional Resources

In addition to the references already listed in this chapter, you may need more information on health insurance, hospitals, or the healthcare system in general. The NIH has set up an excellent guidance Web site that addresses these and other issues. Topics include:[93]

- Health Insurance:
  http://www.nlm.nih.gov/medlineplus/healthinsurance.html
- Health Statistics:
  http://www.nlm.nih.gov/medlineplus/healthstatistics.html
- HMO and Managed Care:
  http://www.nlm.nih.gov/medlineplus/managedcare.html
- Hospice Care: **http://www.nlm.nih.gov/medlineplus/hospicecare.html**
- Medicaid: **http://www.nlm.nih.gov/medlineplus/medicaid.html**
- Medicare: **http://www.nlm.nih.gov/medlineplus/medicare.html**
- Nursing Homes and Long-term Care:
  http://www.nlm.nih.gov/medlineplus/nursinghomes.html
- Patient's Rights, Confidentiality, Informed Consent, Ombudsman Programs, Privacy and Patient Issues:
  http://www.nlm.nih.gov/medlineplus/patientissues.html
- Veteran's Health, Persian Gulf War, Gulf War Syndrome, Agent Orange:
  http://www.nlm.nih.gov/medlineplus/veteranshealth.html

---

[93] You can access this information at:
http://www.nlm.nih.gov/medlineplus/healthsystem.html.

ONLINE GLOSSARIES

The Internet provides access to a number of free-to-use medical dictionaries and glossaries. The National Library of Medicine has compiled the following list of online dictionaries:

- ADAM Medical Encyclopedia (A.D.A.M., Inc.), comprehensive medical reference: **http://www.nlm.nih.gov/medlineplus/encyclopedia.html**

- MedicineNet.com Medical Dictionary (MedicineNet, Inc.): **http://www.medterms.com/Script/Main/hp.asp**

- Merriam-Webster Medical Dictionary (Inteli-Health, Inc.): **http://www.intelihealth.com/IH/**

- Multilingual Glossary of Technical and Popular Medical Terms in Eight European Languages (European Commission) - Danish, Dutch, English, French, German, Italian, Portuguese, and Spanish: **http://allserv.rug.ac.be/~rvdstich/eugloss/welcome.html**

- On-line Medical Dictionary (CancerWEB): **http://www.graylab.ac.uk/omd/**

- Technology Glossary (National Library of Medicine) - Health Care Technology: **http://www.nlm.nih.gov/nichsr/ta101/ta10108.htm**

- Terms and Definitions (Office of Rare Diseases): **http://rarediseases.info.nih.gov/ord/glossary_a-e.html**

Beyond these, MEDLINEplus contains a very user-friendly encyclopedia covering every aspect of medicine (licensed from A.D.A.M., Inc.). The ADAM Medical Encyclopedia Web site address is **http://www.nlm.nih.gov/medlineplus/encyclopedia.html**. ADAM is also available on commercial Web sites such as drkoop.com (**http://www.drkoop.com/**) and Web MD (**http://my.webmd.com/adam/asset/adam_disease_articles/a_to_z/a**). Topics of interest can be researched by using keywords before continuing elsewhere, as these basic definitions and concepts will be useful in more advanced areas of research. You may choose to print various pages specifically relating to merkel cell carcinoma and keep them on file.

Online Dictionary Directories

The following are additional online directories compiled by the National Library of Medicine, including a number of specialized medical dictionaries and glossaries:

- Medical Dictionaries: Medical & Biological (World Health Organization):
  http://www.who.int/hlt/virtuallibrary/English/diction.htm#Medical

- MEL-Michigan Electronic Library List of Online Health and Medical Dictionaries (Michigan Electronic Library):
  http://mel.lib.mi.us/health/health-dictionaries.html

- Patient Education: Glossaries (DMOZ Open Directory Project):
  http://dmoz.org/Health/Education/Patient_Education/Glossaries/

- Web of Online Dictionaries (Bucknell University):
  http://www.yourdictionary.com/diction5.html#medicine

MERKEL CELL CARCINOMA GLOSSARY

The following is a complete glossary of terms used in this sourcebook. The definitions are derived from official public sources including the National Institutes of Health [NIH] and the European Union [EU]. After this glossary, we list a number of additional hardbound and electronic glossaries and dictionaries that you may wish to consult.

Abdominal: Having to do with the abdomen, which is the part of the body between the chest and the hips that contains the pancreas, stomach, intestines, liver, gallbladder, and other organs. [NIH]

ACTH: Adrenocorticotropic hormone. [EU]

Adjuvant: A substance which aids another, such as an auxiliary remedy; in immunology, nonspecific stimulator (e.g., BCG vaccine) of the immune response. [EU]

Anatomical: Pertaining to anatomy, or to the structure of the organism. [EU]

Antineoplastons: Substances isolated from normal human blood and urine being tested as a type of treatment for some tumors and AIDS. [NIH]

Anus: The opening of the rectum to the outside of the body. [NIH]

Apoptosis: A normal series of events in a cell that leads to its death. [NIH]

Aspiration: Removal of fluid from a lump, often a cyst, with a needle and a syringe. [NIH]

Aspirin: A drug that reduces pain, fever, inflammation, and blood clotting. Aspirin belongs to the family of drugs called nonsteroidal anti-inflammatory agents. It is also being studied in cancer prevention. [NIH]

Assay: Determination of the amount of a particular constituent of a mixture, or of the biological or pharmacological potency of a drug. [EU]

Atrial: Pertaining to an atrium. [EU]

Atypical: Irregular; not conformable to the type; in microbiology, applied specifically to strains of unusual type. [EU]

Auditory: Pertaining to the sense of hearing. [EU]

Autologous: Taken from an individual's own tissues, cells, or DNA. [NIH]

Axons: Nerve fibers that are capable of rapidly conducting impulses away from the neuron cell body. [NIH]

Bacteria: A large group of single-cell microorganisms. Some cause infections and disease in animals and humans. The singular of bacteria is bacterium. [NIH]

Basal cell carcinoma: A type of skin cancer that arises from the basal cells, small round cells found in the lower part (or base) of the epidermis, the outer layer of the skin. [NIH]

Benign: Not cancerous; does not invade nearby tissue or spread to other parts of the body. [NIH]

Bereavement: Refers to the whole process of grieving and mourning and is associated with a deep sense of loss and sadness. [NIH]

Biomarkers: Substances sometimes found in an increased amount in the blood, other body fluids, or tissues and that may suggest the presence of some types of cancer. Biomarkers include CA 125 (ovarian cancer), CA 15-3 (breast cancer), CEA (ovarian, lung, breast, pancreas, and GI tract cancers), and PSA (prostate cancer). Also called tumor markers. [NIH]

Biopsy: The removal of cells or tissues for examination under a microscope. When only a sample of tissue is removed, the procedure is called an incisional biopsy or core biopsy. When an entire tumor or lesion is removed, the procedure is called an excisional biopsy. When a sample of tissue or fluid is removed with a needle, the procedure is called a needle biopsy or fine-needle aspiration. [NIH]

Bladder: The organ that stores urine. [NIH]

Bleomycin: An anticancer drug that belongs to the family of drugs called antitumor antibiotics. [NIH]

Bronchial: Pertaining to one or more bronchi. [EU]

Bronchus: A large air passage that leads from the trachea (windpipe) to the lung. [NIH]

Bypass: A surgical procedure in which the doctor creates a new pathway for the flow of body fluids. [NIH]

Calcium: A mineral found in teeth, bones, and other body tissues. [NIH]

Capsules: Hard or soft soluble containers used for the oral administration of medicine. [NIH]

Carbohydrate: An aldehyde or ketone derivative of a polyhydric alcohol, particularly of the pentahydric and hexahydric alcohols. They are so named because the hydrogen and oxygen are usually in the proportion to form water, $(CH_2O)n$. The most important carbohydrates are the starches, sugars, celluloses, and gums. They are classified into mono-, di-, tri-, poly- and heterosaccharides. [EU]

Carboplatin: An anticancer drug that belongs to the family of drugs called platinum compounds. [NIH]

Carcinogenic: Producing carcinoma. [EU]

Carcinoid: A type of tumor usually found in the gastrointestinal system (most often in the appendix), and sometimes in the lungs or other sites. Carcinoid tumors are usually benign. [NIH]

Carcinoma: Cancer that begins in the skin or in tissues that line or cover internal organs. [NIH]

Cardiac: Having to do with the heart. [NIH]

Cardiopulmonary: Having to do with the heart and lungs. [NIH]

Cathepsins: A group of lysosomal proteinases or endopeptidases found in aqueous extracts of a variety of animal tissue. They function optimally within an acidic pH range. [NIH]

Cell: The individual unit that makes up all of the tissues of the body. All living things are made up of one or more cells. [NIH]

Cervical: Relating to the neck, or to the neck of any organ or structure. Cervical lymph nodes are located in the neck; cervical cancer refers to cancer of the uterine cervix, which is the lower, narrow end (the "neck") of the uterus. [NIH]

Cervix: The lower, narrow end of the uterus that forms a canal between the uterus and vagina. [NIH]

Charities: Social welfare organizations with programs designed to assist individuals in times of need. [NIH]

Chemotherapy: Treatment with anticancer drugs. [NIH]

Chloroquine: The prototypical antimalarial agent with a mechanism that is not well understood. It has also been used to treat rheumatoid arthritis, systemic lupus erythematosus, and in the systemic therapy of amebic liver abscesses. [NIH]

Cholesterol: The principal sterol of all higher animals, distributed in body tissues, especially the brain and spinal cord, and in animal fats and oils. [NIH]

Chromosomal: Pertaining to chromosomes. [EU]

Chromosome: Part of a cell that contains genetic information. Except for sperm and eggs, all human cells contain 46 chromosomes. [NIH]

Chronic: A disease or condition that persists or progresses over a long period of time. [NIH]

Cisplatin: An anticancer drug that belongs to the family of drugs called platinum compounds. [NIH]

Colon: The long, coiled, tubelike organ that removes water from digested food. The remaining material, solid waste called stool, moves through the colon to the rectum and leaves the body through the anus. [NIH]

Cryosurgery: Treatment performed with an instrument that freezes and destroys abnormal tissues. This procedure is a form of cryotherapy. [NIH]

Curative: Tending to overcome disease and promote recovery. [EU]

Cytogenetics: A branch of genetics which deals with the cytological and molecular behavior of genes and chromosomes during cell division. [NIH]

Cytoplasm: The protoplasm of a cell exclusive of that of the nucleus; it consists of a continuous aqueous solution (cytosol) and the organelles and inclusions suspended in it (phaneroplasm), and is the site of most of the chemical activities of the cell. [EU]

Dermatologist: A doctor who specializes in the diagnosis and treatment of skin problems. [NIH]

Diarrhea: Passage of excessively liquid or excessively frequent stools. [NIH]

Doxorubicin: An anticancer drug that belongs to the family of drugs called antitumor antibiotics. It is an anthracycline. [NIH]

Dysplasia: Cells that look abnormal under a microscope but are not cancer. [NIH]

Elasticity: Resistance and recovery from distortion of shape. [NIH]

Elective: Subject to the choice or decision of the patient or physician; applied to procedures that are advantageous to the patient but not urgent. [EU]

Emodin: Purgative anthraquinone found in several plants, especially Rhamnus frangula. It was formerly used as a laxative, but is now used mainly as tool in toxicity studies. [NIH]

Enzyme: A protein that speeds up chemical reactions in the body. [NIH]

Epidermal: Pertaining to or resembling epidermis. Called also epidermic or epidermoid. [EU]

Epidermis: The upper or outer layer of the two main layers of tissue that make up the skin. [NIH]

Epidural: The space between the wall of the spinal canal and the covering of the spinal cord. An epidural injection is given into this space. [NIH]

Esophagus: The muscular tube through which food passes from the throat to the stomach. [NIH]

Etoposide: An anticancer drug that is a podophyllotoxin derivative and belongs to the family of drugs called mitotic inhibitors. [NIH]

Extraction: The process or act of pulling or drawing out. [EU]

Extremity: A limb; an arm or leg (membrum); sometimes applied specifically to a hand or foot. [EU]

Fetus: The developing offspring from 7 to 8 weeks after conception until birth. [NIH]

Follicles: Shafts through which hair grows. [NIH]

Gastrointestinal: Refers to the stomach and intestines. [NIH]

Haemodialysis: The removal of certain elements from the blood by virtue of the difference in the rates of their diffusion through a semipermeable membrane, e.g., by means of a haemodialyzer. [EU]

Hybridization: The genetic process of crossbreeding to produce a hybrid. Hybrid nucleic acids can be formed by nucleic acid hybridization of DNA and RNA molecules. Protein hybridization allows for hybrid proteins to be formed from polypeptide chains. [NIH]

Hypothermia: A low body temperature, as that due to exposure in cold weather or a state of low temperature of the body induced as a means of decreasing metabolism of tissues and thereby the need for oxygen, as used in various surgical procedures, especially on the heart, or in an excised organ being preserved for transplantation. [EU]

Immunohistochemistry: Histochemical localization of immunoreactive substances using labeled antibodies as reagents. [NIH]

Immunology: The study of the body's immune system. [NIH]

Implantation: The insertion or grafting into the body of biological, living, inert, or radioactive material. [EU]

Incidental: 1. small and relatively unimportant, minor; 2. accompanying, but not a major part of something; 3. (to something) liable to occur because of something or in connection with something (said of risks, responsibilities, ...) [EU]

Innervation: 1. the distribution or supply of nerves to a part. 2. the supply of nervous energy or of nerve stimulus sent to a part. [EU]

Inoperable: Not suitable to be operated upon. [EU]

Inorganic: Pertaining to substances not of organic origin. [EU]

Interphase: The interval between two successive cell divisions during which the chromosomes are not individually distinguishable and DNA replication occurs. [NIH]

Intravenous: IV. Into a vein. [NIH]

Invasive: 1. having the quality of invasiveness. 2. involving puncture or incision of the skin or insertion of an instrument or foreign material into the body; said of diagnostic techniques. [EU]

Iodine: A nonmetallic element of the halogen group that is represented by the atomic symbol I, atomic number 53, and atomic weight of 126.90. It is a nutritionally essential element, especially important in thyroid hormone synthesis. In solution, it has anti-infective properties and is used topically. [NIH]

Larynx: The area of the throat containing the vocal cords and used for breathing, swallowing, and talking. Also called the voice box. [NIH]

Lesion: An area of abnormal tissue change. [NIH]

Leukemia: Cancer of blood-forming tissue. [NIH]

Liver: A large, glandular organ located in the upper abdomen. The liver cleanses the blood and aids in digestion by secreting bile. [NIH]

Lobectomy: The removal of a lobe. [NIH]

Lymph: The almost colorless fluid that travels through the lymphatic system and carries cells that help fight infection and disease. [NIH]

Lymphoma: Cancer that arises in cells of the lymphatic system. [NIH]

Malignancy: A cancerous tumor that can invade and destroy nearby tissue and spread to other parts of the body. [NIH]

Malignant: Cancerous; a growth with a tendency to invade and destroy nearby tissue and spread to other parts of the body. [NIH]

Mammogram: An x-ray of the breast. [NIH]

Mammography: The use of x-rays to create a picture of the breast. [NIH]

Mechanoreceptors: Cells specialized to transduce mechanical stimuli and relay that information centrally in the nervous system. Mechanoreceptors include HAIR CELLS, which mediate hearing and balance, and the various somatosensory receptors, often with non-neural accessory structures. [NIH]

Mediastinoscopy: A procedure in which a tube is inserted into the chest to view the organs in the area between the lungs and nearby lymph nodes. The tube is inserted through an incision above the breastbone. This procedure is usually performed to get a tissue sample from the lymph nodes on the right side of the chest. [NIH]

Melanocytes: Cells in the skin that produce and contain the pigment called melanin. [NIH]

Melanoma: A form of skin cancer that arises in melanocytes, the cells that produce pigment. Melanoma usually begins in a mole. [NIH]

Melanosis: A disorder caused by a disturbance in melanin pigmentation; melanism. [EU]

Membrane: A very thin layer of tissue that covers a surface. [NIH]

Metastasis: The spread of cancer from one part of the body to another. Tumors formed from cells that have spread are called "secondary tumors" and contain cells that are like those in the original (primary) tumor. The plural is metastases. [NIH]

Metastasize: To spread from one part of the body to another. When cancer cells metastasize and form secondary tumors, the cells in the metastatic tumor are like those in the original (primary) tumor. [NIH]

Metastatic: Having to do with metastasis, which is the spread of cancer from one part of the body to another. [NIH]

Molecular: Of, pertaining to, or composed of molecules : a very small mass of matter. [EU]

Mucosa: A mucous membrane, or tunica mucosa. [EU]

Nasopharynx: The upper part of the throat behind the nose. An opening on each side of the nasopharynx leads into the ear. [NIH]

Nausea: An unpleasant sensation, vaguely referred to the epigastrium and abdomen, and often culminating in vomiting. [EU]

Necrosis: Refers to the death of living tissues. [NIH]

Neoplastic: Pertaining to or like a neoplasm (= any new and abnormal growth); pertaining to neoplasia (= the formation of a neoplasm). [EU]

Nephrectomy: Surgery to remove a kidney. Radical nephrectomy removes the kidney, the adrenal gland, nearby lymph nodes, and other surrounding tissue. Simple nephrectomy removes only the kidney. Partial nephrectomy removes the tumor but not the entire kidney. [NIH]

Nephrology: A subspecialty of internal medicine concerned with the anatomy, physiology, and pathology of the kidney. [NIH]

Neural: 1. pertaining to a nerve or to the nerves. 2. situated in the region of the spinal axis, as the neutral arch. [EU]

Neuroendocrine: Having to do with the interactions between the nervous system and the endocrine system. Describes certain cells that release hormones into the blood in response to stimulation of the nervous system. [NIH]

Neurology: A medical specialty concerned with the study of the structures, functions, and diseases of the nervous system. [NIH]

Neurons: The basic cellular units of nervous tissue. Each neuron consists of a body, an axon, and dendrites. Their purpose is to receive, conduct, and transmit impulses in the nervous system. [NIH]

Nevus: A benign growth on the skin, such as a mole. A mole is a cluster of melanocytes and surrounding supportive tissue that usually appears as a tan, brown, or flesh-colored spot on the skin. The plural of nevus is nevi (NEE-vye). [NIH]

Niacin: Water-soluble vitamin of the B complex occurring in various animal and plant tissues. Required by the body for the formation of coenzymes NAD and NADP. Has pellagra-curative, vasodilating, and antilipemic properties. [NIH]

Non-small cell lung cancer: A group of lung cancers that includes squamous cell carcinoma, adenocarcinoma, and large cell carcinoma. [NIH]

Occult: Obscure; concealed from observation, difficult to understand. [EU]

Octreotide: A drug similar to the naturally occurring growth hormone inhibitor somatostatin. Octreotide is used to treat diarrhea and flushing associated with certain types of tumors. [NIH]

Oncogene: A gene that normally directs cell growth. If altered, an oncogene can promote or allow the uncontrolled growth of cancer. Alterations can be inherited or caused by an environmental exposure to carcinogens. [NIH]

Oncologist: A doctor who specializes in treating cancer. Some oncologists specialize in a particular type of cancer treatment. For example, a radiation oncologist specializes in treating cancer with radiation. [NIH]

Oncology: The study of cancer. [NIH]

Ophthalmology: A surgical specialty concerned with the structure and function of the eye and the medical and surgical treatment of its defects and diseases. [NIH]

Oral: By or having to do with the mouth. [NIH]

Orbital: Pertaining to the orbit (= the bony cavity that contains the eyeball). [EU]

Otolaryngology: A surgical specialty concerned with the study and treatment of disorders of the ear, nose, and throat. [NIH]

Overdose: 1. to administer an excessive dose. 2. an excessive dose. [EU]

Palate: The roof of the mouth. The front portion is bony (hard palate), and the back portion is muscular (soft palate). [NIH]

Palliative: 1. affording relief, but not cure. 2. an alleviating medicine. [EU]

Pancreas: A glandular organ located in the abdomen. It makes pancreatic juices, which contain enzymes that aid in digestion, and it produces several hormones, including insulin. The pancreas is surrounded by the stomach, intestines, and other organs. [NIH]

Pancreatic: Having to do with the pancreas. [NIH]

Pap test: The collection of cells from the cervix for examination under a microscope. It is used to detect changes that may be cancer or may lead to cancer, and can show noncancerous conditions, such as infection or inflammation. Also called a Pap smear. [NIH]

Pathologist: A doctor who identifies diseases by studying cells and tissues under a microscope. [NIH]

Perinatal: Pertaining to or occurring in the period shortly before and after birth; variously defined as beginning with completion of the twentieth to twenty-eighth week of gestation and ending 7 to 28 days after birth. [EU]

Phosphorous: Having to do with or containing the element phosphorus. [NIH]

Potassium: A metallic element that is important in body functions such as regulation of blood pressure and of water content in cells, transmission of nerve impulses, digestion, muscle contraction, and heart beat. [NIH]

Precursor: Something that precedes. In biological processes, a substance from which another, usually more active or mature substance is formed. In clinical medicine, a sign or symptom that heralds another. [EU]

Premalignant: A term used to describe a condition that may (or is likely to) become cancer. Also called precancerous. [NIH]

Prolactin: Pituitary lactogenic hormone. A polypeptide hormone with a molecular weight of about 23,000. It is essential in the induction of lactation in mammals at parturition and is synergistic with estrogen. The hormone also brings about the release of progesterone from lutein cells, which renders the uterine mucosa suited for the embedding of the ovum should fertilization occur. [NIH]

Prostate: A gland in males that surrounds the neck of the bladder and the urethra. It secretes a substance that liquifies coagulated semen. It is situated in the pelvic cavity behind the lower part of the pubic symphysis, above the deep layer of the triangular ligament, and rests upon the rectum. [NIH]

Proteins: Polymers of amino acids linked by peptide bonds. The specific sequence of amino acids determines the shape and function of the protein. [NIH]

Proteoglycan: A molecule that contains both protein and glycosaminoglycans, which are a type of polysaccharide. Proteoglycans are found in cartilage and other connective tissues. [NIH]

Psychotherapy: A generic term for the treatment of mental illness or emotional disturbances primarily by verbal or nonverbal communication. [NIH]

Pulmonary: Relating to the lungs. [NIH]

Radioisotope: An unstable element that releases radiation as it breaks down. Radioisotopes can be used in imaging tests or as a treatment for cancer. [NIH]

Radiologist: A doctor who specializes in creating and interpreting pictures of areas inside the body. The pictures are produced with x-rays, sound waves, or other types of energy. [NIH]

Radiology: The use of radiation (such as x-rays) or other imaging technologies (such as ultrasound and magnetic resonance imaging) to diagnose or treat disease. [NIH]

Radium: Radium. A radioactive element of the alkaline earth series of metals. It has the atomic symbol Ra, atomic number 88, and atomic weight 226. Radium is the product of the disintegration of uranium and is present in pitchblende and all ores containing uranium. It is used clinically as a source of beta and gamma-rays in radiotherapy, particularly brachytherapy. [NIH]

Receptor: A molecule inside or on the surface of a cell that binds to a specific substance and causes a specific physiologic effect in the cell. [NIH]

Rectal: By or having to do with the rectum. The rectum is the last 8 to 10 inches of the large intestine and ends at the anus. [NIH]

Rectum: The last 8 to 10 inches of the large intestine. [NIH]

Recurrence: The return of cancer, at the same site as the original (primary) tumor or in another location, after the tumor had disappeared. [NIH]

Regimen: A treatment plan that specifies the dosage, the schedule, and the duration of treatment. [NIH]

Relapse: The return of signs and symptoms of cancer after a period of improvement. [NIH]

Remission: A decrease in or disappearance of signs and symptoms of cancer. In partial remission, some, but not all, signs and symptoms of cancer have disappeared. In complete remission, all signs and symptoms of cancer have disappeared, although there still may be cancer in the body. [NIH]

Resection: Removal of tissue or part or all of an organ by surgery. [NIH]

Riboflavin: Nutritional factor found in milk, eggs, malted barley, liver, kidney, heart, and leafy vegetables. The richest natural source is yeast. It occurs in the free form only in the retina of the eye, in whey, and in urine; its principal forms in tissues and cells are as FMN and FAD. [NIH]

Screening: Checking for disease when there are no symptoms. [NIH]

Selenium: An essential dietary mineral. [NIH]

Serum: The clear liquid part of the blood that remains after blood cells and clotting proteins have been removed. [NIH]

Skeletal: Having to do with the skeleton (boney part of the body). [NIH]

Somatostatin: A polypeptide hormone produced in the hypothalamus, and other tissues and organs. It inhibits the release of human growth hormone, and also modulates important physiological functions of the kidney, pancreas, and gastrointestinal tract. Somatostatin receptors are widely expressed throughout the body. Somatostatin also acts as a neurotransmitter in the central and peripheral nervous systems. [NIH]

Species: A taxonomic category subordinate to a genus (or subgenus) and superior to a subspecies or variety, composed of individuals possessing common characters distinguishing them from other categories of individuals of the same taxonomic level. In taxonomic nomenclature, species are designated by the genus name followed by a Latin or Latinized adjective or noun. [EU]

Spectrum: A charted band of wavelengths of electromagnetic vibrations obtained by refraction and diffraction. By extension, a measurable range of activity, such as the range of bacteria affected by an antibiotic (antibacterial s.) or the complete range of manifestations of a disease. [EU]

Squamous cell carcinoma: Cancer that begins in squamous cells, which are thin, flat cells resembling fish scales. Squamous cells are found in the tissue that forms the surface of the skin, the lining of the hollow organs of the body, and the passages of the respiratory and digestive tracts. Also called epidermoid carcinoma. [NIH]

Staging: Performing exams and tests to learn the extent of the cancer within the body, especially whether the disease has spread from the original site to other parts of the body. [NIH]

Stomach: An organ that is part of the digestive system. It helps in the digestion of food by mixing it with digestive juices and churning it into a thin liquid. [NIH]

Subcutaneous: Beneath the skin. [NIH]

Systemic: Affecting the entire body. [NIH]

Thermoregulation: Heat regulation. [EU]

Thoracic: Having to do with the chest. [NIH]

Thrombectomy: Surgical removal of an obstructing clot or foreign material from a blood vessel at the point of its formation. Removal of a clot arising from a distant site is called embolectomy. [NIH]

Thrombosis: The formation or presence of a blood clot inside a blood vessel. [NIH]

Thrombus: An aggregation of blood factors, primarily platelets and fibrin with entrapment of cellular elements, frequently causing vascular obstruction at the point of its formation. Some authorities thus differentiate thrombus formation from simple coagulation or clot formation. [EU]

Thyroid: A gland located near the windpipe (trachea) that produces thyroid hormone, which helps regulate growth and metabolism. [NIH]

Thyroxine: An amino acid of the thyroid gland which exerts a stimulating effect on thyroid metabolism. [NIH]

Tomography: A series of detailed pictures of areas inside the body; the pictures are created by a computer linked to an x-ray machine. [NIH]

Toxicity: The quality of being poisonous, especially the degree of virulence of a toxic microbe or of a poison. [EU]

Transfusion: The infusion of components of blood or whole blood into the bloodstream. The blood may be donated from another person, or it may have been taken from the person earlier and stored until needed. [NIH]

Trisomy: The possession of a third chromosome of any one type in an otherwise diploid cell. [NIH]

Tumour: 1. swelling, one of the cardinal signs of inflammations; morbid enlargement. 2. a new growth of tissue in which the multiplication of cells is uncontrolled and progressive; called also neoplasm. [EU]

Unresectable: Unable to be surgically removed. [NIH]

Urine: Fluid containing water and waste products. Urine is made by the kidneys, stored in the bladder, and leaves the body through the urethra. [NIH]

Vaccine: A substance or group of substances meant to cause the immune system to respond to a tumor or to microorganisms, such as bacteria or viruses. [NIH]

Vesicular: 1. composed of or relating to small, saclike bodies. 2. pertaining to or made up of vesicles on the skin. [EU]

Virus: Submicroscopic organism that causes infectious disease. In cancer therapy, some viruses may be made into vaccines that help the body build an immune response to, and kill, tumor cells. [NIH]

Vitiligo: A disorder consisting of areas of macular depigmentation, commonly on extensor aspects of extremities, on the face or neck, and in skin folds. Age of onset is often in young adulthood and the condition tends to progress gradually with lesions enlarging and extending until a quiescent state is reached. [NIH]

Vulva: The external female genital organs, including the clitoris, vaginal lips, and the opening to the vagina. [NIH]

Xenograft: The cells of one species transplanted to another species. [NIH]

General Dictionaries and Glossaries

While the above glossary is essentially complete, the dictionaries listed here cover virtually all aspects of medicine, from basic words and phrases to more advanced terms (sorted alphabetically by title; hyperlinks provide rankings, information and reviews at Amazon.com):

- **The Cancer Dictionary** by Roberta Altman, Michael J., Md Sarg; Paperback - 368 pages, 2nd Revised edition (November 1999), Checkmark Books; ISBN: 0816039542;
  http://www.amazon.com/exec/obidos/ASIN/0816039542/icongroupinterna

- **Dictionary of Medical Acronymns & Abbreviations** by Stanley Jablonski (Editor), Paperback, 4th edition (2001), Lippincott Williams & Wilkins Publishers, ISBN: 1560534605,
  http://www.amazon.com/exec/obidos/ASIN/1560534605/icongroupinterna

- **Dictionary of Medical Terms : For the Nonmedical Person (Dictionary of Medical Terms for the Nonmedical Person, Ed 4)** by Mikel A. Rothenberg, M.D, et al, Paperback - 544 pages, 4th edition (2000), Barrons Educational Series, ISBN: 0764112015,
http://www.amazon.com/exec/obidos/ASIN/0764112015/icongroupinterna

- **A Dictionary of the History of Medicine** by A. Sebastian, CD-Rom edition (2001), CRC Press-Parthenon Publishers, ISBN: 185070368X,
http://www.amazon.com/exec/obidos/ASIN/185070368X/icongroupinterna

- **Dorland's Illustrated Medical Dictionary (Standard Version)** by Dorland, et al, Hardcover - 2088 pages, 29th edition (2000), W B Saunders Co, ISBN: 0721662544,
http://www.amazon.com/exec/obidos/ASIN/0721662544/icongroupinterna

- **Dorland's Electronic Medical Dictionary** by Dorland, et al, Software, 29th Book & CD-Rom edition (2000), Harcourt Health Sciences, ISBN: 0721694934,
http://www.amazon.com/exec/obidos/ASIN/0721694934/icongroupinterna

- **Dorland's Pocket Medical Dictionary (Dorland's Pocket Medical Dictionary, 26th Ed)** Hardcover - 912 pages, 26th edition (2001), W B Saunders Co, ISBN: 0721682812,
http://www.amazon.com/exec/obidos/ASIN/0721682812/icongroupinterna/103-4193558-7304618

- **Melloni's Illustrated Medical Dictionary (Melloni's Illustrated Medical Dictionary, 4th Ed)** by Melloni, Hardcover, 4th edition (2001), CRC Press-Parthenon Publishers, ISBN: 85070094X,
http://www.amazon.com/exec/obidos/ASIN/85070094X/icongroupinterna

- **Stedman's Electronic Medical Dictionary Version 5.0 (CD-ROM for Windows and Macintosh, Individual)** by Stedmans, CD-ROM edition (2000), Lippincott Williams & Wilkins Publishers, ISBN: 0781726328,
http://www.amazon.com/exec/obidos/ASIN/0781726328/icongroupinterna

- **Stedman's Medical Dictionary** by Thomas Lathrop Stedman, Hardcover - 2098 pages, 27th edition (2000), Lippincott, Williams & Wilkins, ISBN: 068340007X,
http://www.amazon.com/exec/obidos/ASIN/068340007X/icongroupinterna

- **Stedman's Oncology Words** by Beverly J. Wolpert (Editor), Stedmans; Paperback - 502 pages, 3rd edition (June 15, 2000), Lippincott, Williams & Wilkins; ISBN: 0781726549;
http://www.amazon.com/exec/obidos/ASIN/0781726549/icongroupinterna

- **Tabers Cyclopedic Medical Dictionary (Thumb Index)** by Donald Venes (Editor), et al, Hardcover - 2439 pages, 19th edition (2001), F A Davis Co.,

ISBN: 0803606540,
http://www.amazon.com/exec/obidos/ASIN/0803606540/icongroupinterna

INDEX

A
Abdominal 74
Adjuvant 13, 14, 104, 106
Anatomical 103
Anus 45, 46, 189, 196
Apoptosis 74, 82, 102
Aspiration 20, 80, 83, 188
Assay 70
Atypical 80
Autologous 145, 157
Axons 100

B
Bacteria 46, 133, 150, 158, 187, 197, 198
Basal 19, 20, 100, 188
Benign 45, 91, 189, 193
Bereavement 35
Biopsy 20, 78, 86, 88, 103, 188
Bladder 66, 198
Bleomycin 145, 157

C
Calcium 151, 152
Capsules 153
Carbohydrate 152
Carboplatin 143, 144, 155
Cathepsins 85
Cervical 33, 45, 180, 189
Cervix 45, 189, 194
Chemotherapy 13, 14, 35, 57, 81, 105, 141, 144, 145, 156
Cholesterol 150, 152
Chromosomal 76, 78, 81
Chromosome 80, 81, 87, 94, 198
Chronic 89, 112, 170
Cisplatin 145, 156, 157
Colon 45, 112, 189
Curative 35, 159, 193
Cytoplasm 102

D
Diarrhea 92, 150, 194
Doxorubicin 145, 157
Dysplasia 71

E
Elective 103
Emodin 145
Enzyme 141
Epidermal 70
Epidermis 20, 91, 100, 102, 188, 190
Epidural 89, 91, 190
Etoposide 143, 144, 155, 156
Extremity 84

F
Fetus 151
Follicles 11, 102

G
Gastrointestinal 21, 87, 91, 188, 196

H
Haemodialysis 144
Hybridization 70, 76, 78, 81

I
Immunohistochemistry 70
Immunology 20, 187
Incidental 90
Innervation 70
Inoperable 141
Inorganic 90
Interphase 81
Intravenous 57, 144, 156
Invasive 125
Iodine 90

L
Lesion 20, 188
Leukemia 112
Liver 11, 21, 90, 98, 101, 152, 159, 187, 189, 192, 196
Lymph .. 11, 12, 14, 45, 72, 73, 78, 82, 85, 86, 88, 100, 102, 103, 104, 106, 189, 192, 193
Lymphoma 79, 112

M
Malignancy 26, 100
Malignant 11, 27, 81, 112
Mammography 32
Melanocytes 21, 45, 71, 192, 193
Melanoma 19, 27, 81, 89, 90, 101, 112
Melanosis 27
Membrane 98, 148, 191, 193
Metastasis 66, 72, 75, 76, 79, 84, 106, 193
Metastasize 21, 26, 192
Metastatic 21, 50, 77, 87, 89, 105, 143, 145, 155, 157, 192
Molecular ... 66, 70, 79, 91, 107, 110, 111, 190, 195
Mucosa 66, 98, 193, 195

N
Nasopharynx 98, 193
Nausea 141
Nephrectomy 193
Neural 70, 92, 151, 192
Neuroendocrine ... 11, 50, 77, 84, 89, 100, 100, 105, 144

Neurons ... 70
Nevus ... 26, 27, 45, 193
Niacin ... 151
Non ... 4, 16, 69, 92, 115, 122, 136, 141, 192

O
Octreotide ... 86
Oncogene ... 92, 112, 194
Oncologist ... 45, 194
Oncology ... 16
Oral ... 158, 188
Orbital ... 72
Overdose ... 151

P
Palate ... 98, 194
Palliative ... 35
Pancreas 21, 45, 79, 90, 91, 93, 187, 188, 194, 196
Pancreatic ... 93, 112, 141, 194
Perinatal ... 71
Phosphorous ... 152
Potassium ... 152
Prolactin ... 50
Prostate ... 35, 91, 112, 135, 140, 141, 188
Proteins .. 78, 91, 126, 133, 150, 152, 191, 196
Proteoglycan ... 87, 156
Pulmonary ... 86

R
Receptor ... 18, 70
Rectum ... 45, 46, 97, 187, 189, 196
Recurrence ... 101, 106
Relapse ... 79

Remission ... 145, 148, 157, 196
Resection ... 104
Riboflavin ... 150

S
Screening ... 28, 35, 54, 56, 59
Selenium ... 152
Somatostatin ... 18, 92, 194
Species ... 21, 94, 196, 198
Spectrum ... 24
Squamous ... 19, 21, 148, 193, 197
Staging ... 12, 26, 102
Stomach ... 90, 91, 93, 98, 187, 190, 191, 194
Subcutaneous ... 101
Systemic ... 13, 98, 103, 189

T
Thermoregulation ... 150
Thrombus ... 197
Thyroid ... 46, 75, 86, 92, 159, 191, 197
Thyroxine ... 152
Tomography ... 79
Toxicity ... 143, 148, 155, 190
Trisomy ... 77
Tumour ... 81

U
Unresectable ... 104, 106
Urine ... 45, 50, 66, 159, 187, 188, 196

V
Vaccine ... 20, 187
Vesicular ... 101
Vitiligo ... 71

X
Xenograft ... 84

Printed in the United States
24410LVS00003B/36